Help!
My Child has
Dyslexia
A Practical Guide for Parents

JUDY HORNIGOLD

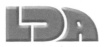

Dedication

I would like to dedicate this book to Sam, for whom every cloud always has a silver lining.

Acknowledgements

I would like to thank Gill Ryland and Adriana Baber for reading the draft copies of this book and commenting so thoughtfully and honestly, my Mum for her proofreading and mastery of the English language and my partner Alan for reading and rereading the text and for his tireless support. I would also like to thank my sons Thomas and James, who have made me endless cups of tea and learned to cook for themselves during the writing of this book. I would also like to thank Bridget Gibbs and Carolyn Jones.

Help! My Child has Dyslexia
ISBN-13: 978-1-85503-503-4
© Judy Hornigold
Inside illustrations: Robin Edmonds (Beehive Illustration)

First published 2011
Printed in the UK for LDA

LDA, Findel Education, Hyde Buildings, Aston Road, Hyde, Cheshire, SK14 4SH

Contents

Chapter 6   A crash course in teaching reading and spelling   59

OVERVIEW
The alphabet
Base words
Suffixes
Prefixes
Syllables
Look for small words within a word
Identify the prefixes and suffixes
Say it wrong to spell it right
Use mnemonics and other memory aids
Identify word families
Answers to questions on page 66

Chapter 7   Games   70

OVERVIEW
Games to improve reading and spelling
Games to improve writing and grammar
Games and techniques to improve memory
Photocopiable templates for games

Final word   92

Useful resources and information   93

Preface

Our family has always loved to read. The house is full of books, so it was no surprise that my twin sons, Thomas and James, also shared a love of reading from a very early age. They would ask for their favourite books repeatedly and in no time at all were picking out words to read for themselves. They soon became fluent readers and read everything that they could lay their hands on. All was going according to plan, but then along came Sam.

Sam clearly had not read the Hornigold child handbook. In fact, he wouldn't and couldn't read anything at all. At the age when Thomas and James had been zooming through the reading stages at school, Sam was literally throwing as many books across the room as tantrums if I tried to help him to read. I couldn't understand what was going on. His behaviour at school was deteriorating and he seemed to be making no progress at all.

Now if any of this sounds familiar to you, then you have come to the right place. This is the book that I wish had been available to me when wooden letters and early readers were being flung across my kitchen on a daily basis.

Dyslexia can have far-reaching effects for the whole family, not just for the dyslexic child. It can be extremely frustrating and very stressful. Nevertheless, there are many things that you can do to make a positive difference to your child's life. A couple of years ago, a grateful parent of a child who was severely dyslexic presented a colleague of mine with an end of term gift. It was a beautiful candle and the card she attached read:

> Thank you for shining a light in a dark place.

I hope that this book goes some way to achieving that light for you and your family.

As for Sam, he is now in secondary school, devouring almost as many books as bars of chocolate and, to quote his own words, has 'got over that dyslexia now'.

Judy Hornigold

About this book

This book has been designed to be an informative and practical resource for busy parents who want to help their dyslexic child.

Each chapter begins with an Overview box, which very briefly summarises the chapter's contents and flags up important points to remember. You can use these boxes, along with the detailed Contents list at the beginning of the book, to find your way around. Also, after you've read the book, dip into the Overviews for a quick reminder of ideas and information that you found particularly relevant or helpful.

An entire chapter has been devoted to games that are easy and fun for you to play with your child and that have been proved to be very successful in supporting their learning. These games can be found in Chapter 7 (page 70), together with photocopiable templates (pages 88–91) to help you make the games at home.

At the back of the book (page 93) there is an extensive resources and information section, which will give you all the support you need to help your child succeed.

Chapter 1

What is dyslexia?

Overview

- Dyslexic children find reading, writing and spelling difficult
- They also have trouble with retrieval of information, memory, processing visual or auditory information, automaticity and organisational skills
- Just as no two children are the same, no two dyslexic children will have the same set of difficulties.

This book will help you to identify exactly what your child is finding difficult and will then show you how you can help.

There seem to be as many definitions of dyslexia as there are dyslexic children. Dyslexia literally means 'difficulty with words'. The dictionary definition of dyslexia is:

> A developmental disorder which can cause learning difficulty in one or more of the areas of reading, writing and numeracy.
>
> *Collins English Dictionary 2009*

The Rose Review, commissioned by the government in June 2009, defined dyslexia as:

> A learning difficulty that primarily affects the skills involved in accurate and fluent word reading and spelling.
>
> *DFES 2006*

Personally, I would define dyslexia as **persistent and unexpected difficulties** in acquiring basic literacy skills. The emphasis here is on the word 'unexpected'. Many children will find it difficult to learn to read, write and spell but dyslexic children have prolonged difficulty that may be unexpected either in relation to their general intelligence or to their development in other areas.

Whichever definition you look at, one thing is clear: dyslexia affects the way that information is processed and this affects the ability to learn.

So what does this mean for your child?

Chapters 1 and 2 of this book will explain the kind of problems that your dyslexic child is likely to face. It may sound all doom and gloom, but take heart, as the rest of the book is devoted to showing you how to help your child overcome these difficulties and how to have fun with them at the same time.

Dyslexic children have many challenges, which may include the following.

Difficulty retrieving information

This relates to our ability to access the information that we have learned and stored in our memory. One way of looking at this is to imagine that your brain is a huge filing cabinet. Everything that you have learned is categorised and neatly filed away. So, when you want to find a piece of information, your brain efficiently locates it and brings it out of the filing cabinet for you.

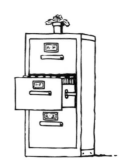

Now imagine that someone comes along and takes all of the files out of the cabinet, throws them up in the air and then dumps them all back into the cabinet in no particular order. Where will your brain go now for a particular piece of information?

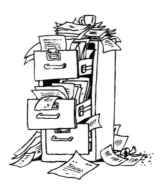

This is what it can be like for many dyslexic children. The information is all there, they just find it very hard to access it.

Sometimes, as adults, we experience this frustrating inability to retrieve information. We just cannot think of a certain word – it is 'on the tip of our tongue' – or we go into a room and cannot think why we went there. For me, this happens with alarming frequency. These episodes can be very irritating, but imagine what it must be like for a dyslexic child, who can face this frustration many times a day.

Poor short-term memory

Poor short-term memory relates to difficulty in storing and working with information. We store information in our memory in different ways. Things that we need to remember all the time, like our telephone number or address, are stored in our long-term memory. Information that we only need to remember temporarily is stored in our short-term memory, which is also referred to as 'working memory'. This is where we store information that we need to use while our brain is working with it.

Many dyslexic children are fantastic at learning new concepts. The problem arises when they cannot transfer this knowledge from their short-term to their long-term memory. To continue the filing cabinet analogy, short-term memory is the information waiting to be filed away, and long-term memory is the information neatly and correctly filed away.

Poor phonological processing skill

'Poor phonological processing skill' means difficulty in forming links between letter patterns (graphemes) and letter sounds (phonemes). Put simply, this means that a child may see the letters sh written together but not be able to link them with the sound sh (as in the word ship). Dyslexic children may hear a word but then be unable to process what they have heard correctly. They cannot translate the sounds they have heard into letters on a page. They may also have trouble in distinguishing individual sounds within words. For example in the word thirsty, they may only be able to distinguish th at the beginning and ty at the end.

Poor visual processing skills

'Poor visual processing skills' refers to the way that our brains process what we see. For example dyslexic children may have difficulty in remembering the sequence of letters in a word because their visual processing skills are impaired. This explains why dyslexic children often write letters and numbers in the wrong order.

Problems with automaticity

Automaticity refers to things that we have learnt so well that we do them without really thinking. Walking is a good example of this! Most of us will have a bank of words that we read and spell so frequently that our brains don't even have to try to remember them any more. Unfortunately, this automaticity of skills can be very hard to attain for some dyslexic children and their brains have to work hard all the time to read and spell even familiar words. This explains why dyslexic children often work at such a slow pace.

Poor organisational skills

Most children find it difficult to plan ahead. If you ask a child to pack the things they need for a holiday at the seaside they would probably come back to you with their swimming costume (no towel ...) and a bucket and spade. The essentials are usually the only things that are on their minds.

With dyslexic children the problem can be even greater as they might not be able to retrieve any items from their memory list of 'things I need at the seaside', or 'things I need to take to school'.

Everyone has their own strategies for organising their lives and for remembering things. I am a list-maker, whereas my teenage son has his world organised on his phone. It is important that your child develops their own strategies that will work for them. This book will help you to find the strategies that might be effective for your child.

Does dyslexia even exist?

At the beginning of this chapter, I referred to the vast number of definitions of dyslexia. This lack of clarity may explain why some people, and unfortunately some schools, refuse to acknowledge dyslexia and put it down either to underachieving children or overanxious parents.

Clearly, some children genuinely struggle to acquire the skills that they need to be competent readers and writers. Now whether you label these children dyslexic or not is, to a certain extent, irrelevant. What matters is that they need extra help and support to acquire these skills and it is up to us as their parents, and up to their teachers, to provide it for them.

I have taught many hundreds of children throughout my teaching career and I can definitely vouch for the fact that dyslexia exists. The problem is that it comes in many different forms and every child will have a different set of difficulties. The skill in helping them is to identify the specific areas that they are finding difficult and to focus on alleviating these particular problems.

Chapters 2 and 3 of this book will help you to identify the areas that your child finds difficult and will show you ways to overcome these problems.

Chapter 2

How can you tell if your child is dyslexic?

Overview

Signs of dyslexia

Most dyslexic children will have some, or maybe all, of the following problems or they might just have problems in one particular area. There is no set pattern of difficulties.

- A marked difference between ability and achievement
- Particular difficulty with spelling
- Difficulty with reading
- Difficulty with writing
- A family history of learning difficulties
- Confusion over left and right
- Reversing letters and numbers
- Difficulty following instructions
- Difficulty with maths.

There is no defined pattern of dyslexia, but there are tell-tale signs. I have detailed below some of these signs of dyslexia. It is important to note, however, that most parents will recognise at least one of these in their children. *This does not mean that they are dyslexic.* For example, letter reversals and left/right confusion are very common in young children. This list is not exhaustive, but if you look through it and recognise several of these traits in your child, then that would be a good indication that they may be dyslexic.

Most dyslexic children will show some, or maybe all, of the signs described on the following pages.

A marked difference between ability and achievement

I would consider this as one of the best indicators of dyslexia. It is also one that is easily missed. Some dyslexic children are highly intelligent and develop strategies to cope with their difficulties. I remember Sam telling me to stop worrying that he could not do the work at school because he could 'just copy from the person sitting next to him'. These children can appear to be doing fine at school and often fall under the radar, so they are not flagged up for special attention. The crucial point here is the difference between what they *should be* achieving and what they *actually are* achieving.

For example if your child is very bright then you would expect them to be reading, writing and spelling at a level above their chronological age. So a very able 7 year old may be expected to have a reading age of 9 or 10. However, they may only be achieving a reading age of 7. Parents and teachers may not pick up this discrepancy between ability and achievement because the child is reading at a level appropriate for their age. The problem is that they are not reading at a level appropriate for their *ability*.

Frequently, a very able child will perform well verbally and will typically have a broad vocabulary, but will not translate this into their written work.

You may find this scenario familiar.

Parent: Have you thought up your story for homework yet?

Child: Yes. It is brilliant. Charlie and I went down to the park on our bikes. It was getting dark and out of the corner of our eyes, we saw a ghost-like figure appearing through the woods. It approached us with a menacing stare and we heard a loud and low groaning. Charlie and I were terrified and rode home at supersonic speed.

Parent: That's fantastic. Now go and write it in your book.

Quite a while later, having employed many delaying tactics and with many crossings out, your child comes back with their book. They have written:

I whent to the parck on my bik and plade with Charlie. We sor a gost. Then went home.

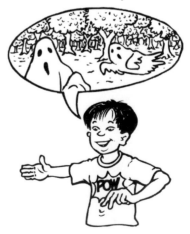

Particular difficulty with spelling

Spelling is the one area that many dyslexic children find the most difficult. They will often have several attempts at a particular word and will usually make one or more of the following mistakes.

✿ Spelling words as they sound: 'phonetic spelling'

Phonetic spelling works well for some words that are spelt as they sound, for example **bat** and **dog**. However, many English words are not spelt as they sound. Words like **could** and **though** can be very tricky if you try to spell them by sounding out individual letter sounds.

Currently there is a strong emphasis on phonics in schools and, generally, this is an excellent way of teaching a child to read, but dyslexic children like to cling on to a rule or a particular structure and then apply it to everything they come across so they may end up writing:

> **wos** for **was**

and

> **sed** for **said**.

This type of phonetic spelling is common in children who are just learning to read and write, up to the age of 6 or 7. However, these problems may persist in dyslexic children for many years. I have come across several children who still struggle to spell words like **was** and **said** in secondary school.

✿ Bizarre spellings

Dyslexic children will often invent their own bizarre spellings. This is particularly true if they also have hearing or phonological processing difficulties.

For example **kum** may be written for **come** and my son, Sam, once inventively wrote **at most fear** for **atmosphere**.

✿ Inconsistent spelling

Words may be spelt correctly at the start of a piece of writing only to be misspelt later on. This can be particularly frustrating for a parent, because you think that your child has mastered a particular spelling only to find that they have spelt it incorrectly later on in their writing.

✿ Incorrect letter order

Many dyslexic children have trouble with sequencing, which in turn will lead to problems with spelling, as they cannot remember the correct order for the letters in a word or they process them out of order.

Therefore, they may spell **tame** as **team** or they may see the word **verse** but read it as **serve**.

Word order may also be confused, where a child may read **are we** instead of **we are**.

This has obvious implications for how well a child will understand what they are reading. If they are reading words incorrectly then it is quite likely that the sentence won't make any sense at all.

✂ Omitting letters or adding extra letters

Some children find it very hard to isolate the individual sounds in a word. For example in the word **find** they may not be able to hear the **n** sound so will write **fid**.

Alternatively, they may insert extra letters, commonly putting an extra **e** before **y** at the end of a word, for example writing **maney** for **many**.

✂ Inability to say if a word 'looks right'

When spelling a tricky word, we will often look at the word to see if it 'looks right'. We are using our visual memory here as we search to find a familiar look for a word. For example we may look at the word **becoz** and know that it does not look right: **oz** is not a spelling pattern that is commonly used at the end of English words. Dyslexic children often have poor visual memory, so do not have the ability to judge whether a word 'looks right' or not. They will 'sound out' the word **becoz** and might think that it is a perfectly acceptable way to spell **because**.

Difficulty with reading

Many children will find learning to read difficult, but dyslexic children will typically have the following problems.

✂ Difficulty blending letters together

One of the basic building blocks of reading is the ability to blend sounds together. For example **c- a- t** says **cat**. If a child has difficulty blending sounds then they will find it very hard to work out how to read a new word. This skill is typically acquired between 4 and 6 years of age.

✂ Difficulty using the 'look and say' method

The 'look and say' method of learning to read is used for words that are not spelt the way they sound. Words like **come** and **said** will be taught using the 'look and say' method. Children will be presented with the word on a flashcard and the child will have to learn that word by sight.

✿ Difficulty splitting words into syllables

Reading is made much simpler if you can split a word into syllables. For example the word **computer** can be split into **com- pu- ter**, three syllables that are individually quite easy to read.

If a child finds it hard to split long words into syllables, then it will be very hard to read them correctly.

✿ Adding or missing out words when reading

You might notice when your child is reading aloud that they add extra words or miss words out completely. They might add words because they are guessing what the text is likely to say or because they cannot read a particular word and are substituting their own words. They might miss words out simply because they can't read them or because they have lost their place on the page.

✿ Inconsistency in reading

In a similar way to spelling, there may be inconsistency in what can and can't be read. A word might be read correctly on one page but incorrectly on the next. This might be because your child is using picture or context clues to help them to read a particular word. These clues may be present on one page of the text but not on another page. Note that using picture and context clues is a strategy to be encouraged and is an important tool that we all use when reading. However, your child will also need to be able to read words out of context and in isolation.

✿ Poor understanding of what has been read

This is not surprising, since if your child is struggling to read most of the words on a page then they will find it very hard to keep up with the meaning of the text.

Difficulty with writing

Trying to persuade your dyslexic child to write can be an incredibly frustrating experience. You will discover just how ingenious your child can be in diversionary tactics and they may even turn on a bit of emotional blackmail for good measure. These avoidance strategies are all basic items in the dyslexic child's tool kit and will be devices that have been born out of necessity for many of them. It is amazing how many times Sam needed the toilet when we were doing some writing.

I have detailed below some of the difficulties that your child may be facing. They might not have all of them, so it would be a good idea to highlight the areas that you feel apply to your child. Then you can focus on these areas when you are writing with them.

✿ Inability to translate their verbal skills into writing

As I mentioned earlier, dyslexic children often have a lot to say but then find it almost impossible to put this down in words.

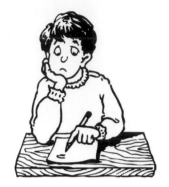

- They may not know how to start
- They may be unable to order their thoughts in a logical way
- They may have difficulty with finding the right words
- They may take an inordinately long time in thinking what sentences to write
- Their ideas may be confused, with no planning or structure.

✿ Poor handwriting

Quite often, dyslexic children will have poor motor control, which means that they will find it hard to control a pencil, leading to untidy and spidery handwriting.

✿ Poor understanding of basic punctuation

Typically, they will write everything in one long sentence sprinkled with dozens of **ands**, no capital letters and no full stops.

This is an example written by a child in Year 8:

> england were going to win the match and someone tackled him and he was injured and the person who tackled was sent off and then germany scored and they won.

If your child writes like this, ask them to read it back to you. Tell them they can only take a breath if they see a comma or a full stop. It will highlight the problem quite effectively.

✿ Bizarre spelling

As mentioned earlier, spellings tend to be phonetic and you may only be able to decipher what your child has written by reading it aloud.

✿ Many words crossed out

To compound the untidy handwriting, there will be frequent crossing outs as children try different versions of spellings.

✿ Overuse of displacement activity

This is something that we all do. How many times have you been about to settle down to something that you don't really want to do, maybe the ironing or cleaning the cooker, and thought 'I will just phone my friend first', or 'I'll just have a cup of tea before I get started'? Well, as I am sure you have experienced, children are masters of this art and dyslexic children are world leaders. They will use every trick in the book to avoid writing, from frequent toilet breaks to pencil sharpening and endless anecdotes about their friends or what they have been watching on television.

✿ Tiring easily

Since writing is such a difficult activity for dyslexic children, it is no surprise that they will tire easily. They will become fidgety, bad tempered and even tearful after what we consider a relatively short space of time.

A family history of learning difficulties

Frequently, but not always, there will be a family history of learning difficulties. It may be that one parent has dyslexic-type difficulties, although the person may not have been acknowledged as being dyslexic when they were at school.

Confusion over left and right

Many children find this difficult. A friend of mine had a jumper with the words *left*, *right*, *front* and *back* strategically placed on it when she was 16; and she wasn't dyslexic.

We talk about children being left handed or right handed. This also applies to the feet, the ears and the eyes. Most people will favour either the left side or the right, but dyslexic children can favour a mixture of these. For example a dyslexic child may be right handed, but left footed and right eyed. This is called cross laterality and can be a cause of both left/right confusion and letter reversals.

If you want to find out if your child has cross laterality, it is quite simple.

✿ Left/right handed

I expect you know this already. It is the hand that they will use to pick up a pen to write.

✿ Left/right footed

Put a ball on the ground in front of your child and ask them to kick it. Do this at least twice and make sure the ball is in the middle, not directly in front of one of their feet. Make a note which foot they use to kick the ball.

✿ Left/right eyed

Make a tiny peephole in a piece of paper and then put it on a table in front of your child. Ask them to pick up the paper and look through the peephole. Make a note of which eye they use to look through the peephole.

✿ Left/right eared

Put a ticking watch on the table and ask your child to put it to their ear to hear it tick. Make a note of which ear they hold the watch to.

If your child favours a mixture of left and right then this may indicate dyslexia.

Reversing letters and numbers

This is a common problem for any young child. It is no surprise as the letters c, a, o, d, g, q, e, f, s all start on the right and flow to the left, as do the numbers 5, 6, 8, 9 and 0, but the numbers 2, 3, 7 start on the left and flow to the right, as do the letters m, n, u, v and w. You will find that children generally reverse the numbers 2, 3 and 7.

Also, the letters b and d are frequently confused. This is such a common problem that there are many books and games aimed at tackling this confusion.

Most children get over this quite quickly, usually by the time they are 7, but if your child is persistently reversing letters and numbers then this may be an indication that they are dyslexic.

Difficulty following instructions

Dyslexic children can find it very hard to remember complex instructions. For instance, imagine the following classroom scene.

> Alice, can you go to the office, ask for the dinner register and find out whether Mrs White is coming into school today. Also, can you ask Mr Davies if I can borrow his stapler. Thanks, Alice!

This type of instruction is far too complicated, as it requires both memory and sequencing skills and it is very unlikely that Alice will come back with the register, the stapler and the information about Mrs White.

Most children love being given jobs to do but dyslexic children need much simpler direction. A more appropriate request would be:

> Alice, can you go to the office to collect the dinner register?

Difficulty with maths

Not all dyslexic children have difficulty with maths, but those that do tend to have trouble with the following areas.

✿ Difficulty with sequencing numbers and in identifying number patterns

In exactly the same way that dyslexic children will muddle up letters in a word, so they can also muddle up the sequence of digits in a number.

✿ Transposing numbers

For example: writing 21 for 12 or confusing + and ×.

✿ Difficulties remembering times tables

Learning the times tables relies heavily on remembering sequences.

✿ Difficulties using mathematical language

Mathematical language is not very dyslexia-friendly. Terms like 'numerator' and 'denominator' in fractions, and 'acute' and 'obtuse' in angles, can be very difficult for a dyslexic child to read and understand.

✿ Difficulty solving word problems

Word problems can also cause real difficulties, as much of the information may be irrelevant in terms of finding a solution, but the child still has to plough through it all to find out how to solve the problem. Your child may be perfectly capable of completing the mathematics involved, but they run out of time as it has taken them so long to decipher the words.

Chapter 3

What you can do to help your child

Overview

Helping with spelling
- Practise phonetic spelling
- Use pure sounds
- Teach spelling patterns
- Use 'mobile memory'
- Use mnemonics
- Use magnetic tiles/Scrabble™ tiles
- Look for words within words
- Illustrate the words
- Play games with word cards

Helping with reading
- Find something that interests your child
- Find books that are part of a series
- Use audio books
- Watch television (with the subtitles on)
- Set up a book group

Reading techniques
- Blend letters together
- Use 'look and say' games for irregular words
- Split words into syllables
- Read aloud or tape your child reading
- Highlight tricky words

Ways to improve comprehension
- Active reading
- Use the TELLS technique
- Use the PQ4R method

Helping with writing
- Write about something that interests your child
- Use different writing formats
- Use a variety of pens and paper, a whiteboard or a laptop
- Scribe for them
- Create a family newsletter
- Provide story starters
- Write a plan
- Use word banks
- Encourage proof-reading

Helping with maths
- Teach 2, 3, 7 separately from 5, 6, 8, 9, 0
- Use auditory and visual memory games
- Use the finger method for tables
- Use a highlighter for word problems
- Use mobile memory for mathematical words.

Chapters 1 and 2 have highlighted the problems and difficulties faced by dyslexic children and could make depressing reading for even the most resilient parent! This chapter aims to show you how you can address these problems and will go some way to explaining why your child has these difficulties. Each of the difficulties highlighted in Chapters 1 and 2 are covered below, with ideas and suggestions for ways in which you can help your child to overcome them.

Helping with spelling

✂ Phonetic spelling

Don't be put off by the terms 'phonetic or 'phonic'. They just refer to 'sound'. Therefore, with this method, sounds are put together to make up a word. Many words in English are spelt phonetically so this is a good place to start.

Every letter in the alphabet has both a name and a sound.

For example:

> The name of the letter *a* is pronounced *a* as in *acorn*.
> The sound of the letter *a* is pronounced *a* as in *apple*.

When using the phonic method, children will sound out all the letter sounds in a word and then join, or 'blend', them together to make the word.

For example:

> *f- o- g* when blended will say *fog*.

It is vital when using this method that you only use 'pure sounds'. It is very tempting when sounding out words to add the sound 'uh' at the end.

For example:

> sounding *c- a- t* as 'cuh' 'a' 'tuh'.

This can lead to a great deal of confusion for a young child trying to blend sounds together.

It can be tricky to isolate the pure sounds but the best way is to say out loud a word beginning with the sound that you want and then say it out loud again but without the ending.

So, to find the pure sound for *l* say *lamp* and then say it again without the *amp*.

It does become easier with practice! I have listed out the alphabet on page 24 so that you can practise isolating the pure sounds of all 26 letters.

✿ Pure sounds

a say **at** without the **t**   n say **nut** without the **ut**
b say **bed** without the **ed**   o say **odd** without the **dd**
c say **cat** without the **at**   p say **pen** without the **en**
d say **dog** without the **og**   q say **quick** without the **ick**
e say **egg** without the **gg**   r say **red** without the **ed**
f say **fish** without the **ish**   s say **sun** without the **un**
g say **gate** without the **ate**   t say **tap** without the **ap**
h say **hat** without the **at**   u say **up** without the **p**
i say **it** without the **t**   v say **van** without the **an**
j say **jam** without the **am**   w say **wet** without the **et**
k say **king** without the **ing**   x say **box** without the **bo**
l say **lamp** without the **amp**   y say **yes** without the **es**
m say **man** without the **an**   z say **zip** without the **ip**

✿ Bizarre spellings

Your child might invent bizarre spellings. For example they might write:

heyer for **here**

or

pleez for **please**.

This is generally because they are trying to spell non-phonetic words in a phonetic way. However, if you read the word aloud then you will usually be able to unravel what your child is trying to say. The way to help your child to avoid using these bizarre spellings is to teach them the common spelling patterns for these tricky words.

For example **tion** is the most common way of spelling **shun** in words. Therefore, once this pattern has been learnt then your child will stop writing **stashun** for the word **station**.

Try to teach spellings in 'word families'. Choose between five and ten words with a particular spelling pattern and work with these until your child has learnt them. A list of common word families is given in the resources and information section on pages 97–104.

For example if you are working on the **ing** pattern, you could give your child the following words:

bring, cling, fling, king, ring, sing, sting, thing, wing

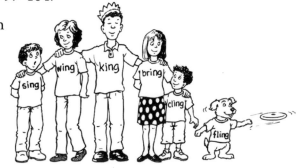

In Chapter 7, there are many ideas for games and activities for you to play with your child for any list of words that you are working on. One of these games is Noughts and Crosses, as illustrated below.

Noughts and Crosses

bring	wing	cling
fling	sting	thing
sing	king	ring

 You will need:

A board of nine squares, with one target word written in each square.

A wipe-clean board is perfect for this. Once your child has mastered the words you can simply wipe them off and write in your new set of target words.

Two sets of coloured counters – or a few 1p and 5p coins.

 How to play

Player 1 takes a counter or coin and reads one of the words on the board. If they have read it correctly then they can place their counter over the word. Once they have covered the word the player will then have to spell the word. If the word is spelt correctly, the counter stays on. If spelt incorrectly, it is removed.

Player 2 now has their turn.

The first player to cover three words, horizontally, vertically or diagonally is the winner.

✿ Inconsistent spelling

The reason why dyslexic children are inconsistent in their ability to spell is that frequently they have poor working memory. Your working memory is where you store information temporarily while you are working with it.

To explain this concept further, imagine that you want to write the following sentence.

I ran to the bus station.

You will need to retrieve the spelling patterns for all these words from your long-term memory and store them in your working memory while you write the sentence. Once you have written the sentence the words can leave your working memory, as you don't need them any more.

Dyslexic children may have problems:

- Retrieving the words from their long-term memory
- Storing these words for any length of time in their working memory
- Transferring a word from short-term to long-term memory.

So what can you do to help them improve their memory?

Dyslexic children need to 'overlearn' new words. This means that they will need to revisit the same information many times to make sure that they have transferred this new knowledge from their short-term to their long-term memory.

This sounds like a major task, but actually spending just five to ten minutes every day can make a huge difference and will be much more effective than one long session once a week. Little and often is the key to success.

✿ 'Mobile memory'

This is a very effective way to help your child to remember new words. Write the words that your child is learning onto small business-sized cards. Buy a business card box or wallet to keep them in. Spend a few minutes every day practising reading and spelling these words. Once they are secure in your child's memory, leave one example of the spelling pattern in your card box and then move on to the next set that you want to work on.

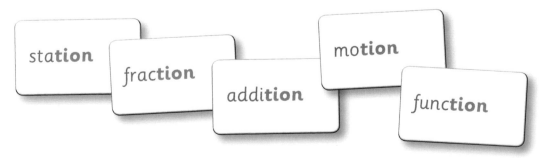

✢ Incorrect letter order, omitting letters or adding extra letters

Dyslexic children often have problems with sequencing. This is due to problems with auditory and visual memory.

⊙ Auditory memory

Auditory memory is the ability to hear a sequence and to remember it in the correct order. A child may ask how to spell the word **right** and the response would be **r-i-g-h-t**. If the child has good auditory memory, they will remember the correct sequence of these letters when they come to write the word. Dyslexic children often have poor auditory memory and cannot remember the correct sequence of letters.

Games to improve auditory memory are detailed in Chapter 7, the games chapter of this book. However, one quick method is outlined below.

Alphabet Rainbow

 You will need:

A set of wooden or plastic letters.

 How to play

Ask your child to set out the letters in alphabetical order in a rainbow shape.

Now select four letters at random. Tell your child that you are going to give them four letters to find.

For example you may say

      G   X   C   M

Your child has to:
1 Remember this list.
2 Select the letters from the rainbow in the order that you said them.

You can make this game harder by increasing the number of letters that they have to remember and by using distraction. This means that you give them the list to remember and then ask them to do something else, such as run up and down the stairs, or 'put your shoes in your bedroom'. If you are canny about this, you could get them to do no end of little jobs while you are playing this game! When they come back, they have to remember and select the letters, but this time it is harder as they have had time to forget.

☺ *Visual memory*

Visual memory is the ability to remember a sequence that we have seen in the correct order. In the above example, if the word right is written out for the child, then providing that they have good visual memory they will be able to go away and write the word correctly from memory. This can be very hard for dyslexic children, as they cannot keep an accurate picture of the correct letter order in their memory.

The Alphabet Rainbow, as described on page 27, can be equally useful in improving visual memory. The method is exactly the same but instead of saying the letters aloud, you write them on a card and show them to your child. More ideas for games to improve visual memory can be found in Chapter 7.

✿ Inability to say if a word 'looks right'

Many of us rely on our visual memory when it comes to spelling a word. We decide if the word 'looks right'. Children with poor visual memory will find it very hard to tell if a word 'looks right'. Visual memory can be improved through repetition. The more times a child sees a particular word then the more they are likely to be able to rely on their visual memory for that word. This is why schools use flashcards for words that are difficult to spell, and why children who love reading tend to be good at spelling. They have come across the word so many times that they have been able to store the word in their long-term visual memory.

Flashcards on their own are not a particularly dyslexia-friendly resource, but can be very useful when incorporated into games. See Chapter 7 for suggestions for using flashcards.

Other strategies to help with spelling

✿ Mnemonics (pronounced 'nemonics')

This peculiar (and totally dyslexia-unfriendly) word provides an excellent way of helping children to spell tricky words.

Take each letter in the word and use these letters as the initial letters of a silly saying or phrase.

For example:

BECAUSE = Big Elephants Can Always Upset Small Elephants

Encourage your child to think up their own mnemonics, as this will help them to remember them, and the sillier the better as not only will this aid their memory but it also makes it more fun.

✿ Magnetic tiles/Scrabble™ tiles

Using a set of letter tiles, give your child all the letters that they need to spell a word and ask them to put the letters in the right order.

For example for the word *again* you will give them *a a g i n*.

Using this method will harness your child's motor memory (also called kinaesthetic memory) and is a valuable way of helping them to learn tricky spellings.

✿ Look for words within words

See if you can find smaller words hidden within the word. (Note that you must not change the letter order.)

For example:

heart

In the word *heart* are the words

he, hear, ear, art

In the word *comfortable* are the words

for, fort, or, tab, table, able

The process of finding and writing out these words will ensure that your child will always remember how to spell the words *heart* or *comfortable*.

Sentences can be made linking the smaller words to the original word.

For example:

piece

The word *pie* is hidden in the word *piece*.

So you could make the sentence:

Can I have a piece of pie?

✿ Illustrate the words

If your child is artistic then they could illustrate the words.

Children are more likely to remember a word that has a picture associated with it.

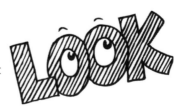

✿ Homophones

Homophones are words that sound the same but are spelt differently, for example **here** and **hear**. They can cause all sorts of problems and are best learned through association with pictures. A list of common homophones can be found in the resources and information section on pages 109–112.

Helping with reading

One major problem with reading for dyslexic children is boredom. They often find that the books they are able to read have a content that is not interesting or appropriate for their age group.

Some publishers, such as Barrington Stoke, are now addressing this issue. They have an excellent range of books that are high interest, written in an easy to read format, for different levels of reading ability. For more details, see www.barringtonstoke.co.uk

As I mentioned in the introduction to this book, with my first two children, reading was never a problem. With my third child, Sam, it was a very different story. He resisted reading at every opportunity. He loved being read to, and would often ask for the same story again and again... and again. However, he hated reading his school reading book and we had many tears and tantrums as I tried in vain to spark his enthusiasm for reading.

In the end, the Simpsons saved the day. Having previously decided that this was not suitable viewing for my impressionable young child, through sheer desperation and exhaustion, I ended up letting him watch every episode and bought him the Simpsons comic every month. It was the only thing that he would actually read. This in turn led to him starting to read other comics and as he became more confident, his love for reading did grow and now at the age of 12 he, at last, will read for pleasure.

If the Simpsons don't work for you then joke books and nonsense poems are a good place to start. They tend to be short and are intrinsically high interest because they are funny. However, reading material is all around us, so you are sure to find something that interests your child. If they like football then encourage them to read the football programmes from the matches or if they like shopping ask them to read shop names and advertising hoardings.

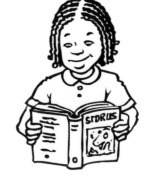

My advice, therefore, is to let them read whatever they want. Find something that interests them and then exploit it for all it is worth. You, like me, may have to turn a blind eye to the content.

Other strategies to encourage reading

✂ Find books that are part of a series

If your child enjoys a particular author, they will want to read more. Therefore, books that come in a series will naturally encourage them to read more.

I have listed series of books that are particularly useful for reluctant readers in the resources and information section on pages 133–136.

✂ Use audio books

When choosing books for your child try to find the audio book version as well as the actual book. Make sure that it is the unabridged (word for word) version. These can be expensive but most libraries have a good selection. Then let your child listen to the audio version as well as reading the book. The familiarity with the story that they gain from the audio book will help them to read the book for themselves. This in turn will help them to build confidence in their reading, and they will enjoy the book even more.

How you use these audio books will depend on how well your child can read the actual book.

If they are struggling then try following the book as the audio plays in the background.

If they are becoming more confident, then get them to listen to a chapter first and then read it without the audio version.

Then as they become more competent, they can read a chapter and just listen to the audio version to reinforce their comprehension of the text.

✂ Watch television

When your child is watching their favourite programme put the subtitles on. This will help them to read, as even subconsciously they will be processing the words on the screen together with the sounds from the television. To start with, you could have the volume running alongside the subtitles but you could also try it with the volume off. This will be a very strong motivation for them to read (and will give you some peace and quiet). However, this should only be used if they can read most of the words.

✂ Consider setting up a book group

This is more suitable for older children, around 10 years old and above, and you will need to be careful that your child is not surrounded and intimidated by more fluent readers. However, if carefully managed it can be a fun way for your child to enjoy reading as well as spending time with their friends.

The children can each suggest a book to be read over the course of two or three weeks. Then they can meet up and talk about what they liked or disliked about the book. You will soon find that children will start recommending books to each other and this is a great way for them to expand their reading. They are much more likely to read something that a friend has recommended rather than something their parents have recommended.

Reading techniques

There are many different techniques that you can use to teach your child to read. Chapter 6 is entitled 'A crash course in teaching reading and spelling' and will give you more detail but, in short, the following methods are used.

✿ Blending letters together

Previously, when looking at how children spell we looked at pure sounds. These are the sounds that you will need to use when you blend letters together. The pure sounds are explained on page 24.

Some words blend by only using individual letters.

For example:

The word **bed** can be read by blending together the sounds *b- e- d*.

Some words blend by using a combination of individual letters and consonant blends or digraphs.

Consonant blends are a combination of two or three consecutive consonants. Each individual sound can be heard.

Digraphs are two or more letters that join together to make a new sound.

Consonant blends that appear at the beginning of words are:

br bl cl cr dr fl fr gl gr pl pr sc scr sk sl sm sn
sp spr st str sw tr

The word **trip** can be read by blending the sounds *tr- i- p*.

Consonant blends that appear at the end of words are:

-ct -ft -ld -lf -lk -lm -lp -lt -mp -nd -ng -nk -nt -pt
-sk -sp -st

The word **left** can be read by blending the sounds *l- e- ft*.

Digraphs that appear at the beginning of words are:

ch ph sh th wh

The word **chip** can be read by blending the sounds ch- i- p.

Digraphs that appear at the end of words are:

-ch -ck -sh -tch -th

The word **bench** can be read by blending the sounds b- e- n- ch.

✺ Using the 'look and say' method

Below are listed 100 or so words that represent half the words that we most frequently use in reading and speaking. Therefore, if your child can master the reading and spelling of these words then they will have learnt 50 per cent of the words that we use the most. Some of these words are spelt phonetically but many are irregular words, which need to be learnt using 'look and say' or other methods.

☉ *Phonetically spelt words*

These are much easier to learn and you can use the blending method.

a, an, and, at, back, big, but, can, did, from, get, had, has, him, his, if, in, is, it, just, must, not, of, off, on, up, well, went, will

☉ *Irregular words*

These words are harder and you will need to be more inventive about learning them.

about, all, are, as, be, been, before, by, call, came, come, could, do, down, first, for, go, have, he, her, here, I, into, like, little, look, made, make, me, more, much, my, new, no, now, old, one, only, or, other, out, over, right, said, same, see, she, so, that, the, their, them, then, there, they, this, to, two, want, was, we, were, what, when, where, which, who, with, you, your

✺ Suggestions for ways to learn irregular words

☉ *'Look and say' games*

Chapter 7 is full of ideas for teaching your child how to read and spell these irregular words. Games like Snap, Pairs and Happy Families can all be easily adapted using word cards.

One such game, called Post It, is described on page 34.

Post It

You will need:

A set of cards with about ten irregular words written on them.

A posting box (I use the small cylindrical crisps tubs, washed and covered with red paper, with a posting slot cut into the plastic lid – but any box with a slit cut into one side will do).

How to play

Lay the cards face up on the table. Your child has to read a card to be able to post it into the post box. You can make this harder by setting a time limit.

The post box will also serve as a good place to store your cards while you are not using them.

| again | about | here | after | there |

⊙ *Splitting words into syllables*

Longer words need to be broken down into sections that are more manageable.

A syllable is a beat in a word. All syllables will have a vowel sound in them.

For example the word **escalator** has four syllables. As it stands, **escalator** would be quite a hard word to read, but when it is broken down into syllables then it becomes much easier:

es- cal- a- tor

Being able to split words into syllables is an invaluable skill for any dyslexic child. Most dyslexic children have a limit to the number of pieces of information that they can remember at any one time. Imagine that their working memory is a small bookshelf. There is room on the shelf for three or maybe four books. When you try to put another book on the shelf then one of the original books will fall off. This is what it can be like for children trying to read and spell long words. By the time they get to the end of the word they have forgotten what came at the beginning.

In our example with the word *escalator*, splitting words into syllables has reduced the pieces of information that need to be recalled from the nine individual letters of *escalator* to just four syllables.

✿ What to do if your child is adding or missing out words

Dyslexic children will often add or miss out words when they read. They frequently read what they think is there on the page and not what is actually there.

Reading aloud can help with this problem, or you and your child could take it in turns to read a word each.

Another idea is for your child to tape their own voice as they read aloud and then follow the text again as they play back the tape. They should be able to spot where they have missed or added words.

✿ Developing consistency in reading

It can be very frustrating to find that your child reads a difficult word on one page only to read it incorrectly later on. One way to help with this problem is to take a highlighter pen and highlight the tricky words in the text. Clearly, you won't be able to do this with school or library books, but if you have access to a photocopier or scanner you could make a copy of the page. By highlighting the problem word, you are focusing your child's attention on that word and they are more likely to read it correctly every time. If they keep making mistakes, then incorporate it into your list of words to be learned through games.

✿ Understanding what has been read

Quite often, your child will have taken so long to read a passage that they have lost all sense of what the passage was about.

This can be a real problem for dyslexic children. If they don't understand what they have read, they have put in all that effort for nothing. Here are a few ideas to improve reading comprehension.

Ways to improve comprehension

✿ Active reading

What does active reading mean?

Have you ever read a page of a book and realised at the end that you have not taken in a single word? Generally, this happens because we have been distracted by thinking about something else and although our eyes are reading the words, our brain is not processing any of the information. We have not been *actively involved* in the process of reading.

There are several techniques that you can use to encourage your child to be a more active reader.

1 Before you open the book

Look at the title and the front cover.

> What clues do these give you about the story?
> Read the blurb on the back.
> What do you think may happen in the story?

2 On the first page, look for the heading

Make sure that your child gets into the habit of looking for and reading headings. You would be amazed how many children ignore them.

3 Read the first page

If your child is struggling then help them with the more difficult words to keep the flow of reading going.

If they are struggling with more than 10 per cent of the words, then the book is too hard and you will need to find something simpler.

If your child gets tired, then you and your child can take it in turns to read a sentence, a paragraph or a page each.

Books that are in play script form are great for sharing with dyslexic children as you, your child and other family members can all take on different parts. Children's poetry is also excellent, as it tends to be a bit silly or even rude.

4 Question as you read

What has happened so far?
Why has this happened?
What do you think might happen next?
What do you want to happen next?

5 When you finish the book

Try and recall the main events.
Did your child enjoy the book?
If so, why and if not, why not?

As your child becomes older and more confident you can encourage them to use this technique when they read independently.

I would recommend two versions of active reading: the **TELLS technique** for younger children and **PQ4R** for older children.

✂ The TELLS technique

This has been proven to be very effective for younger children. It was developed by Idol-Maestas in 1985.

TELLS is an acronym for:

*T*itle
What is the title? It sounds obvious, but the title is often overlooked. The title will give the children information about the text and will help them to locate their memory store of information about that topic.

*E*xamine
Look through each page of the story and skim pages for clues. Look at the illustrations, the paragraph headings and any tables or diagrams.

*L*ook for important words
Find out what they mean if your child doesn't already know.

*L*ook for hard words
Try to split these words into syllables to make them easier to read.

*S*etting
What is the setting of the story? When and where did it take place? Is the story fact or fiction?

Just spending a few minutes going through these stages will improve your child's comprehension immensely.

✂ PQ4R technique

A more detailed method suitable for older children who are reading information texts is called the PQ4R method.

PQ4R stands for Preview, Question, Read, Reflect, Recite and Review. (There are four steps that begin with R, hence PQ4R.)

*P*review
Look at the heading and the sub-headings, and read the first paragraphs of each section, as these will give you the main ideas in the text. Look at the illustrations, diagrams and captions to give you further information.

Question

Question yourself about what you have learned in the preview. What do you think the main points of the text are? What are you expecting to learn? Are there areas that you don't understand that you will need to concentrate on as you read the text?

Read

Read the passage carefully and make notes in the margin, if you can, or on paper. Be careful not to write out great chunks of text. Notes are just meant to be key words or key points.

Reflect

Reflect on what you have read with someone else. Did you understand it? What have you learnt? Are there any areas where you are still unsure?

Recite

Discussing what you have read with someone else is a great way to help you remember it and also to make sure that you understand it.

Review

What were the main points of the text? Have you any questions still to be answered?

Helping with writing

Getting your dyslexic child to write is likely to be one of the hardest things that you will have to do. As I mentioned in Chapter 2, you have a bit of a mountain to climb here but, as with any long journey, it starts with a single step.

My advice would be not to think about reaching the summit in one go, but rather to take a few steps every day and little by little you will start to make inroads in your journey. Make sure you rest and regroup at the camps regularly before tackling the next section of the climb!

Remember, you will need to have vast reserves of patience. Be kind to yourself and try to share the load with other adults if possible. Don't expect too much too quickly but take time to celebrate your child's achievements, however small they may be.

So here are a few ideas for helping your child to write.

✿ Write about something that interests your child

Sometimes you just have to accept that your child's choice of subject matter may not be the one that was top of your list. You may prefer that they write about the wonderful trip you had to the museum last week and how much they learned while they were there, and they may want to write about the boy at school who was sick all over the dining table and how it got into everyone else's lunch boxes.

In fact, the subject matter is not important at all. What matters is that your child is writing.

✿ Use different writing formats

Use postcards, cartoons, speech bubbles, shopping lists, labels and so on. Try to make the writing part of another activity that your child enjoys. So if they like computer games get them to write a wish list of games that they would like. Letter writing is also an excellent way of encouraging your child to write, especially if you can get willing family and friends to write back, as all children love to receive letters in the post. This will also encourage their reading, as they will want to read the letters that they receive.

✿ Use a variety of pens, paper and white boards

White boards are great as your child can 'write and wipe' to their heart's content and you won't be left with reams of waste paper. Dry wipe pens are widely available in a variety of colours.

✿ Use a laptop

Although using a laptop will not help your child's handwriting, it will help them to develop their writing skills. Children can have lots of fun experimenting with different fonts and colours. There are also some excellent software programmes for teaching your child to touch type. For details, see the list of websites in the resources and information section on pages 137–140.

✿ Magic pens

There are pens available now that will erase ink. These can be great for dyslexic children of secondary age, as they can correct their work without having to cross things out.

✿ Scribe or type for them

Although this won't help if you do it all the time, it definitely has its place. It is particularly useful for creative writing as your child will be able to let their imagination run wild without the constraints of being limited to words that they can spell correctly.

✿ Create a family newsletter

If you or a member of your family is computer literate, then publishing a family newsletter can be a great way to involve everyone in writing. Each member of the family will need to produce an article about something that they have done or learnt during the week.

✿ Provide story starters

Even the most prolific author can suffer from writer's block at some time. Therefore, it can really help your child to give them a sentence or two to start them off. This technique is frequently used in schools.

✿ Write a plan

Writing a plan can really help your child to focus their thoughts. It will provide structure for your child and stop them from wandering off the point.

✿ Use a word bank

Providing your child with a word bank is a great way to support their writing.

For example: If they have to write a scary story you could provide them with a list of useful words, such as:

> dark, horrible, creepy, screech, shadows, monstrous
> (and so on)

Word banks can be provided for any topic and are useful for children of all ages.

✿ Proof-reading

After your child has finished their piece of writing, then encourage them to go back over it, as if they were the teacher, and highlight any words that they think may be spelt incorrectly. You can also ask them to read it aloud and this should highlight basic punctuation they may have missed.

✿ Don't stress about the spelling

This may seem to be a strange piece of advice, but if your goal is to encourage your child to write then you will have to be relaxed about their spelling. They are not going to want to be inventive with vocabulary if every time they make a spelling mistake they have to correct it. So, if your child's spelling is poor, then it can be best to ignore most of the spelling errors. Otherwise, you could risk stopping their flow of writing. If writing is the task, then spelling can take a back seat. This is particularly true if they are word processing, as they can always spell check their work afterwards.

The games chapter of this book, Chapter 7, will also provide you with many ideas and activities to stimulate your child's writing.

✿ Confusion over left and right

One easy way to remember this is to hold up your hands with the fingers together and your thumbs sticking out towards one another. Your left hand will make the shape of a capital L.

✿ Confusion over b and d

Make cards with these pictures on to help your child to remember which way round b and d go.

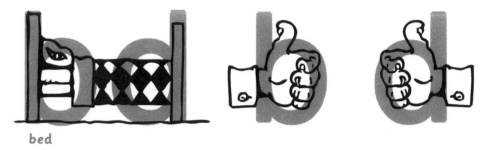

bed

Helping with maths

✿ Reversing numbers when they write

You will need to teach numbers in two separate groups.

- ⊙ *Group 1*
  2, 3, 7 start on the left and move towards the right.

- ⊙ *Group 2*
  5, 6, 8, 9, 0 start on the right and move to the left.

Young children will enjoy writing these numbers in sand trays, or in the air with their fingers, or using paints. Brushes dipped in water can be used to 'paint' the numbers onto paving slabs in the garden.

The numbers can also be made with playdough or clay. You could even use real dough and bake bread numbers!

Much of the work that you do to improve auditory and visual memory will have a positive impact on any difficulties that your child has with mathematics, particularly with sequencing and reversals.

✿ How to help with the times tables

2 × table: This is one of the easiest to remember, as all the numbers are even numbers:

>   2, 4, 6, 8, 10, 12, 14, 16, 18, 20, 22, 24

5 × table: All of the numbers in this table end in a 5 or a 0:

>   5, 10, 15, 20, 25, 30, 35, 40, 45, 50, 55, 60

10 × table: All of these end in 0:

>   10, 20, 30, 40, 50, 60, 70, 80, 90, 100, 110, 120

9 × table: Use the finger method – see below.

>   9, 18, 27, 36, 45, 54, 63, 72, 81, 90, 99, 108, 120

4 × table: Just double all the answers to the **2 ×** table:

>   4, 8, 12, 16, 20, 24, 28, 32, 36, 40, 44, 48

11 × table: up to 9 × 11 this follows a nice pattern as all the answers are just the number written down twice:

>   11, 22, 33, 44, 55, 66, 77, 88, 99 then 110, 121, 132

So this just leaves us with the 3 × table, the 6 × table (which is just double the 3 × table) the 7 × table and the 8 × table.

The 7 × and 8 × tables are the hardest, but most of these can be worked out from the other tables.

The three that you just have to learn are:

>   a) 7 × 7 = 49
>   Wakey wakey rise and shine, 7 × 7 is 49

>   b) 7 × 8 = 56   (56 = 7 × 8)
>   You can remember this as they are in number order: 5, 6, 7, 8.

>   c) 8 × 8 = 64
>   I ate and I ate till I could pick no more
>   ('pick no more' sounding like 'sixty four').

✿ The finger method – for the 9 × table

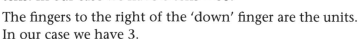

Put both your hands up in front
of you as shown here.

Mentally number your fingers 1–10
from left to right.

To find out 7 × 9, put your seventh
finger down.

The fingers on the left of this are the
tens. In our case we have 6 tens = 60.

The fingers to the right of the 'down' finger are the units.
In our case we have 3.

Add the tens and the units. 60 + 3 = 63.

So we have discovered, using only our fingers, that:

$7 \times 9 = 63$

This will work for the 9× table up to 9 × 10.

✿ What to do about mathematical language

Use the 'mobile memory' technique by building up a
bank of cards with the particular words that your child
is working with. Use mnemonics and pictures to help
them to remember what the word means. The bigger,
bolder and sillier the pictures the better.

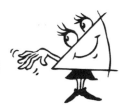

A 'cute' angle

✿ How to solve word problems in maths

The key to answering these questions is to recognise what information is
relevant. Use a highlighter to highlight the important bits.

Follow these steps:

1 Read the word problem at least twice.
2 Highlight key words that are maths related. For example words such
  as **altogether**, **total**, *difference*, *how many*, and so on, will give you
  clues as to how to work out the answer.
3 Highlight the important numbers and write these down on the answer
  sheet.
4 Decide what mathematical operations to use. Is the question asking
  you to multiply, divide, add or subtract?
5 Estimate what you think the answer will be. This only has to be a
  rough estimate.
6 Work out the answer to the problem.
7 Check your answer against your estimate. Does it make sense?

Chapter 4

What are learning styles?

Overview

Learning styles
There are eight different learning styles. The three main ones are:

- Visual – learning through seeing
- Auditory – learning through hearing
- Kinaesthetic – learning through doing.

Find out your child's dominant learning style and use that to help them.

Make sure that you encourage your child to use all three learning channels when they are working with you or playing the games.

Help to build their self-esteem on a daily basis.

We all learn from listening, looking, saying and doing. But we have different ways in which we prefer to learn new things and these are our individual learning styles.

To illustrate this, think about an occasion when you have visited a museum or an exhibition. Do you prefer to read all the information, or do you prefer to listen to the audio guide, or do you prefer to interact with the exhibits and go round pressing all the buttons and making things happen?

- If you prefer to read then your learning style is **visual**. You favour learning with your eyes.

- If you prefer to listen then your learning style is **auditory**. You favour learning with your ears.

- If you prefer to interact and touch things then your learning style is **kinaesthetic**. You favour learning with your hands.

There are actually eight different types of learner, but the main ones are visual, auditory and kinaesthetic. Understanding your child's learning style can provide you with the key to how they learn most effectively and can also give you an insight into why they are having difficulties at school.

What is your child's learning style?

Read the following statements with your child and tick all the ones that apply to them. Then count how many ticks they have for each style. You will probably find that your child has ticks in more than one style.

✿ Visual

I remember things better if I write them down	
When I think of spellings I picture them in my head	
I have to look at someone when they speak to me	
I find it difficult to concentrate when there's a noise	
I like looking at maps and pictures	
I am not very good at remembering jokes	
I like to doodle and make notes when I learn something new	
I am good at thinking of ideas in my head	
I remember people's faces	
I like to make lists	
When I get a new idea I like to write it down or draw a picture	
I learn a practical skill best by watching someone do it	
I love doing crosswords and word searches	

Total number of ticks for visual [ ]

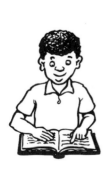 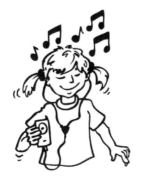 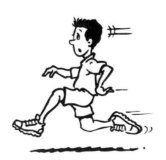

✿ Auditory

I remember things better if I hear them	
I like to discuss things before I start to work	
I work better if I'm not alone	
I would rather hear new things than read about them	
I sometimes look out of the window even though I am listening	
I don't like working on more than one task at a time	
I love telling jokes	
I remember people's voices	
I like learning the words of songs and rhymes	
I like reading and writing poetry	
I find it hard to picture things in my head	
I like reading out loud	
I remember things by 'hearing' them in my head	

Total number of ticks for auditory

✿ Kinaesthetic

I hate listening to instructions – I'd rather have a go	
I don't like sitting still	
I use my hands to describe things	
I like to walk around when I'm working	
My desk looks messy to everyone else but I know where things are	
I like to talk out loud when I'm working	
I like to work on projects and designing things	
I don't mind noise when I work	
I like to plan my work in my head before I begin	
I hate checking my work after I have finished	
I sometimes take notes but I never use them	
I like to act and do drama	
It sometimes takes me a while to get started on a new project	

Total number of ticks for kinaesthetic

You can find these tables online at http://www.keystageplus.co.uk/learningstyles.pdf (© Learn4life Publishing Ltd 2007).

Once you have identified your child's learning style, it is important to try to develop the other styles. This is to help your child access information in as many different ways as possible and also to help them when they come across a teacher whose style is different from their own.

So how do we develop other learning styles and how do we make the most of our child's preferred learning style?

Ways to help kinaesthetic learners

37 per cent of children will be kinaesthetic learners. This is the most common preference for learning.

An old Lakota proverb sums it up beautifully:

Tell me	I will listen
Show me	I will understand
Involve me and	I will learn

Kinaesthetic learners remember what they do, more than what they see or hear.

If your child is a kinaesthetic learner then make sure you use the following techniques when working with them.

⚙ Flashcards

These are widely used in schools, but need to be used in short sharp bursts with not too many cards in a pack.

For example if you were looking at the **tion** ending with your child you could write ten words with this ending on ten separate business-card-sized pieces of card.

I would either highlight the letters **tion** or write them in a different colour.

For example: sta**tion**

These cards can now be used for reading practice, where the child has to read the word, or for spelling practice, where you say the word and the child writes it down – preferably without looking at the card!

✿ Post it® notes

These are a great way of helping your kinaesthetic learner to organise themselves. They don't have to worry too much about spelling or grammar and can just jot down what they need to remember (for example *Need PE kit for Weds*) and stick it onto their desk, homework book, fridge and so on.

✿ Strips of paper

This is where a 'Blue Peter' training will come in handy. We are now entering the world of sticky back plastic and coloured paper!

Simple sentences can be written on strips of paper and then cut up into words for your child to rearrange. You could highlight the nouns, verbs and adjectives (see Glossary page 141) for your child by colour coding them.

> *The / greedy / dog / ran / away / with / the / juicy / sausages.*

✿ Letter tiles

These are invaluable when teaching a kinaesthetic learner to spell. The tiles from a box of Scrabble™ will do or if you have a few hours to spare (unlikely I know), then you could make your own set. I have a set that I have printed onto magnetic paper so that they can be used on a magnetic board or even on the fridge door.

There are three main ways of using these for spelling.

1 Give the child the correct letters that they will need to spell a word and ask them to put them in the right order. For example for the word *Wednesday*, give them *a, e, e, d, d, n, s, w, y* and ask them to spell out *Wednesday*.
2 Ask them to select the letters they need to spell *Wednesday*. If they make a mistake don't correct them until they have discovered it for themselves. Or, if they are happy with their spelling but it is wrong then help them to find out for themselves where they have gone wrong.

   For example if they spell *Wednesday* as *Wensday*, then tell them that they need two more letters, one vowel and one consonant.
   Keep on giving clues until the child gets it right.
3 Once your child has correctly spelt the word ask them to break it up into chunks. For example:
   Wed nes day.

For a word like **Wednesday** it is a good idea to over pronounce it. I call this 'saying it wrong to spell it right'. So you would pronounce it **Wed- nes- day**.

✿ Games

All children love games, but this is especially true for kinaesthetic learners. As this makes up such a large part of this book, Chapter 7 is an entire chapter devoted just to games.

✿ Fidgeting

For obvious reasons this is discouraged in schools where a whole class of children is trying to learn, but at home there is no reason why your child can't learn while walking around or standing up. Many of my dyslexic students prefer to stand rather than to sit. My mother used to learn Latin verbs by running up and down the garden reciting them to herself.

Ways to help auditory learners

34 per cent of children will be auditory learners. This means that they learn by listening and also by explaining to others what they have learned.

This is the predominant style of teaching in the United Kingdom. The teacher talks and the children listen (most of the time at least!). So here is where problems may lie. Nearly 40 per cent of children are kinaesthetic learners but the majority of teachers are auditory teachers.

However, many teachers today will try to vary their teaching styles, as they understand that most children prefer to be involved rather than just to listen.

Peer tutoring is also a valuable tool that teachers use. This can involve one child explaining something to another child. You can use this method quite easily with your child by asking them to explain something to a sibling, a friend or even a pet. There is nothing quite like explaining something to someone else to find out if you really understand it yourself. As a slightly rusty teacher of A level maths, I can tell you that there have been occasions when I could truly vouch for that theory.

When working with auditory learners, make sure that your sessions are noisy. Encourage your child to always say things aloud.

✿ Mnemonics

We first met mnemonics in Chapter 3 and they are a great way for auditory learners to harness their memory.

For example: **said** – take each letter in turn and think of a word that begins with that letter.

Silly Ants In Doughnuts

It works best if the child has thought up their own words and the sillier the image they create the better. This will make it easier for them to remember how to spell the word.

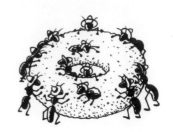

The mnemonic can be written on a card and the children can illustrate it on the reverse.

Word of warning! Some children absolutely love these and can remember them perfectly. However, they lose their value if the child is being overloaded with words to remember and then forgets which words they needed. So use them sparingly for the trickiest of words.

As you make your own mnemonics, you will find that elephants and octopuses can come in very handy.

These are just two examples:

COME: Come On My Elephant

SOME: Some Octopuses Move Everywhere.

✿ Storytelling

Storytelling is another way to help auditory learners to remember. If you have a list of words to remember, you and your child can make up elaborate and fanciful stories that contain all of your target words. This way, they are more likely to remember them. Alternatively, you could take a well-known story, such as Jack and the Beanstalk, and retell it trying to get all your target words into your version.

Ways to help visual learners

29 per cent of children are visual learners. This means that they prefer to learn by looking at things.

Visual learners respond well to diagrams, charts and mind maps. They love to have things colour coded.

Visual learners hate to be dictated to and prefer to have a sheet of writing in front of them for them to annotate and colour code.

When using mnemonics the visual learner will remember the word from the picture that they have drawn.

Other learning styles

✿ Mathematical learners

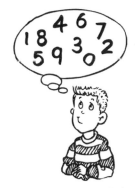

These children are very logical and methodical in their approach. They enjoy solving problems. This style of learning is a valuable one as it works well with the three main styles: auditory, visual and kinaesthetic.

✿ Musical learners

Being able to recognise rhyme and rhythm in words can be a powerful tool for any learner, but particularly for a dyslexic learner. Children find it easier to remember things in rhymes or songs, which is why a lot of early learning is done through nursery rhymes.

For example:

> 1, 2, 3, 4, 5
> Once I caught a fish alive
> 6, 7, 8, 9, 10
> Then I let him go again.

Clearly **five** rhymes with **alive**, and **ten** rhymes with **again** (although in the latter the spellings are not the same).

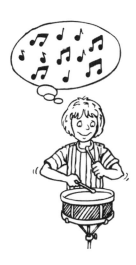

Dyslexic children, like all children, will be able to recite the words to their favourite songs easily and this is a skill that we can harness for other areas of learning.

Having music playing in the background can also help these children to focus and to remember.

✿ Social learners

These children like to learn with other children. They are generally confident in presenting their ideas to a group or class of children and enjoy taking on the role of supporting other members of a group.

In my experience, most dyslexic children prefer to work in isolation for fear of their mistakes being made public.

✿ Intuitive learners

These children prefer to work on their own. Many dyslexic children will fall into this category although they may not have the same sense of internal motivation that intuitive learners tend to have.

✿ Emotional learners

I believe this is the most important learning style. Children may be visual, auditory or kinaesthetic learners but it is highly desirable for them to be strong emotional learners as well.

These children have positive self-esteem and are happy to face new challenges as they have gained confidence from being successful in the past. They learn from their mistakes and don't become discouraged by them.

We would all want our children to be confident with high self-esteem, but sadly, this is unlikely to be the case for many dyslexic children. Some children have had their confidence shattered by too many experiences of failing. To build self-esteem it is vital that these children are working well within their comfort zones before we ask them to move on to more challenging things.

Imagine being asked to do something that you know you are going to fail at. For me, at school, it was gymnastics. I absolutely hated it. I couldn't do it and would go to great lengths to try to avoid it. I felt that I was the only person in the class who could not do it and I was convinced that the other children were laughing at me. It was not a pleasant experience but, fortunately, it only happened once a week.

For dyslexic children the scenario is much worse. They are asked several times a day to do things that they can't do, while watching children around them achieving the same task with apparent ease. Whether it is reading, spelling or writing they are constantly being reminded of their inadequacies. Is it any wonder that they have low self-esteem?

This is the hardest part of all for the parent of a dyslexic child but it is vitally important. It takes a very long time to build up a child's confidence but it can be destroyed in an instant.

How to build your child's self-esteem

1 Be honest. Your child will know if you are praising them for anything and everything regardless of whether it is any good or not, and then your praise will be meaningless.

2 Find the positive in all that they do. Even if they present you with a piece of writing that is littered with mistakes, there will be something positive to say about it. They may have improved their handwriting, or they may have used interesting vocabulary.

3 Praise them to the heavens for the skills that they do have. Many dyslexic children are creative or good at sports, so find something that your child can do really well and give them the chance to shine.

4 Be patient. You may find that your child's progress seems incredibly slow. They may learn something one day and forget it the next. They may even be able to read a particular word at the beginning of a passage but not at the end. This is normal for dyslexic children, as they find it hard to transfer knowledge from their short-term to their long-term memory.

5 Keep smiling. You may be feeling frustrated but this is nothing compared with the frustrations that your child is facing on a daily basis.

6 Give them opportunities to succeed. Try to present your child with games and activities that you know they will be able to succeed at. This is tricky as you don't want to demotivate them by giving them things that are babyish or boring, so they need to have an element of challenge but they also need to be within your child's comfort zone. This book is full of ideas to help you to achieve this. So read on!

The key here for helping your child is patience, and you will need it by the bucket load.

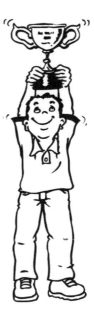

Chapter 5

Multisensory teaching and learning

Overview

- Use multisensory methods
- Have one-to-one time
- Little and often is the key
- Mistakes are good
- Always give praise
- Make it fun!

In Chapter 4, we looked at the different learning styles that children can have and acknowledged that teachers will also have different teaching styles. It can be difficult for a visual learner to learn effectively from an auditory teacher.

One way of overcoming this problem is to teach in a multisensory way and to encourage the child to learn in a multisensory way. So what exactly does this mean and how does it work?

Multisensory simply means using many senses, namely sight, sound and touch.

Therefore, if you are helping your child to learn how to spell a word then they will be more likely to remember it if it has been taught in a multisensory way. This is because the messages to the brain are coming through several channels, not just one.

For example imagine if you had to learn how to spell **always** just by being told how to spell it. All you have had is auditory input.

Therefore, you cannot see the word and you haven't experienced how it feels to write the word or say the word.

Now imagine that you can see the word, you read it, you say it aloud, you say the sound of each letter and you write out the word. Now, your brain has had a lot more information about this word and you are much more likely to be able to remember it.

Currently, most schools use a look, cover, write, check approach to spelling, in which the child looks at the word, covers it up, writes it from memory and then checks it.

This activity can be made more multisensory – and therefore more effective – by saying the word aloud as you look at it, and then saying the letters as you write them, and then saying them again as you check the word.

Specialist dyslexia teachers will always teach in a multisensory way. So lessons can become quite noisy.

This is a simple yet particularly effective way for you to help your child. It will also help to develop the learning styles that they may not be particularly strong in. When working with your child or when playing the games in this book with them, try when possible to make sure that you are doing it in a multisensory way.

Specialist teaching

Specialist teaching can have a huge impact on your dyslexic child's learning. While it is not possible within the constraints of this book to train you to be a specialist teacher, I can give you an insight into how it is done and offer you a few strategies to use at home with your own child.

Many practitioners are very wary of parents teaching their own children and similarly many parents avoid this for fear of 'doing it wrong'. There is also the question of the parent/child relationship being far more emotional and complicated than the teacher/child relationship.

Personally, I have no end of patience with the pupils that I teach but get frustrated very quickly with my own children. Teaching your own child is not always an easy path to tread, but if you approach it in the right way and with the right tools and techniques at your fingertips you can make a real difference to your child and also have some fun time together along the way.

These are the some of the main techniques that specialist dyslexia teachers will use.

One-to-one lessons

All children love to have one-to-one attention. Even if the one-to-one time is a lesson in a subject that they are really struggling with, they will still enjoy the attention. This is something you can do as a parent with no special training at all. However, you will need a little preparation beforehand. Make sure that you are in a quiet room 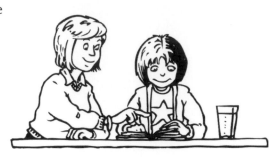 alone with your child and free from distractions. You will both need to be comfortable, not hungry or thirsty or tired. Have all the equipment that you will need to hand and set a time limit for the session. Finally, always reward your child at the end even if just with a cuddle or a sticker. I used marbles in a glass jar with Sam, so that he could see his collection growing after every session. He was always keen to fill the jar as this meant that he would have a larger treat such as a new computer game or a trip out.

One of the areas that is likely to hold dyslexic children back at school is a lack of confidence. They will be reluctant to put their hand up in class for fear of appearing stupid. Therefore, if they don't understand something then the chances are that they will continue not to understand it.

However, in a one-to-one situation they will be able to ask anything they like safe in the knowledge that they are not going to be ridiculed. I have seen many of my own pupils mouth silently the answer to a question before saying it aloud. So even in a safe and secure environment they are rehearsing their responses just to make sure they don't feel silly by making a mistake.

Children hate to make mistakes in front of others but one-to-one teaching can show them that:

> Mistakes are good!

It can be very liberating for your child to understand that mistakes are good! This is not the way that they will have seen the world before. Yet, making mistakes is the way that we learn. If we are challenging ourselves to achieve a higher goal then we are going to make mistakes. It is a vital part of the learning process. So let them know that mistakes are good. They are an integral part of the way we learn.

Logical, structured, cumulative approach

Learning to read and write is very much like building a house. The alphabet is the foundation upon which everything else is built and each stage of the building has to be secure and well-formed before the next stage is tackled. You can't put the roof on until you have built the walls.

So specialist teachers will use a very structured step by step approach, in which one lesson will lead on to the next, gradually getting a little more complicated as you go along.

Repetition and short sharp bursts

Little and often is definitely my motto. It is far better to spend ten minutes on activities with your child every day than to spend one hour once a week.

I usually illustrate this point with the idea of walking through a field of tall grass. You are the first person to walk across this field and as you do so, your footsteps make a pathway through the field. Then you go back the following week and the grass has bounced back and your pathway has disappeared.

However, what if you revisited that field every day for a week and walked the same pathway? On the second day, you can just make out where your pathway was, so you can go over it again. On the third day, the pathway is even clearer and by the end of the week, it is a clear track that will remain and one that you can revisit whenever you like.

This is exactly how your memory works. You need to revisit information several times before it is transferred from your short-term memory into your long-term memory.

Dyslexic children can find it very hard to make this transfer, and that is why we think they have learned something only to find that a few days later they have forgotten it.

Praise

Every child likes to be praised, just as every child likes to have one-to-one attention. Even if your child is really struggling, there will be something that you can praise. They may have:

- Listened well
- Remembered how to spell a tricky word
- Remembered capital letters/full stops
- Tried hard with their handwriting
- Sounded out the letters correctly
- Or even beaten you in a game!

There will always be something positive. The skill is in spotting it and using praise as a means to motivate your child and to build their self-esteem. This is not always easy and there have been times when Sam and I have both been on the verge of tears, but even then there would always be something positive. Even it was only that he had not thrown the book across the room.

Making it fun

Not many of us would choose an activity that we found difficult as a way of spending our leisure time. As interesting as it would be, I would not choose to spend my evenings learning how to write Chinese characters. It would be too hard and exhausting after a busy day. I am much more likely to go for a walk in the countryside or put my feet up in front of *Coronation Street*.

So spare a thought for your dyslexic child, who has just spent another frustrating day at school, being presented with tasks that they find difficult at best and impossible at worst. Then they get home and you say 'Right. It's time to go over your spellings and finish your reading book'. They will probably start moaning, complaining of headaches, feeling too tired, or needing the toilet, and so on. All the avoidance and diversion tactics at their disposal will come into play.

The best approach is to give them some down time and to make your sessions short and fun. The more that you can make it into a game, the more they will learn and the less they will realise that they are learning.

The next chapter is entitled 'A crash course in teaching reading and spelling' and will give you some idea of how English words are constructed.

Chapter 6

A crash course in teaching reading and spelling

Overview

The terms used

(See also the full Glossary on pages 141–143.)

The alphabet

The alphabet is made of 26 letters.

Vowels

The five vowels are **a, e, i, o, u.** Vowels have two sounds: a short sound and a long sound.

Consonants

There are 21 consonants in the alphabet.

Consonant blends

Consonant blends are two or more consonant letters, whose sounds blend, with each individual sound retaining its identity.

Digraphs

Digraphs are two or more letters that join to make one sound.

Base words

This is an original word, before any suffixes or prefixes have been added.

Suffixes

A suffix is a letter or group of letters added to the end of a base word to change its use or meaning.

Prefixes

A prefix is a group of letters added to the beginning of a base word to change its meaning.

Syllables

Syllables are beats in a word. Each syllable has a vowel sound.

Strategies

- Split words into syllables
- Look for small words within a word
- Identify the prefixes and suffixes
- Say it wrong to spell it right
- Use mnemonics and other memory aids
- Identify word families.

So, let's start at the beginning. We need to look at some terminology and definitions first. Try not to be put off by all this terminology. The main idea is for you to understand how words are built so that you can split them successfully into smaller meaningful chunks.

Basically, you are learning how to build them so that you can knock them down.

The alphabet

The alphabet is made of 26 letters. Five of these are vowels and the rest are consonants. Of course, as in life, nothing is ever that simple and the consonant **y** sometimes acts like a vowel. In words like **cry** it sounds like an i and in words like **happy** it sounds like an e.

cry – y sounds like i

happy – y sounds like e

y can also appear as a vowel in the middle of a word such as **style**, **pyramid** or **dynamite** where it makes an i sound.

✿ Vowels

The five vowels are:

a, e, i, o, u

Vowels have two sounds: a short sound and a long sound.

1 Short sounds

a as in **apple**
e as in **egg**
i as in **ink**
o as in **octopus**
u as in **umbrella**

Short vowel sounds can be distinguished in words by using a symbol called a breve. A breve looks a bit like a smile and is written above the vowel to show that it is making a short sound.

For example:

căt

2 Long sounds

These are the letter names.

a as in *alien*

e as at the start of *evening*

i as in *ice cream*

o as in *open*

u as in *unicorn*

Long vowel sounds can be distinguished in words by using a symbol called a macron. A macron looks like a long line and is written above the vowel to show that it is making a long sound.

For example:

āble

✿ Consonants

There are 21 consonants in the alphabet but in the same way that vowels can be long and short, some consonants, namely c and g, can be hard or soft.

c can be hard as in *cat* where it makes a k sound

c can be soft as in *ceiling* where it makes an s sound

g can be hard as in *go* where it makes a g sound

g can be soft as in *gentle* where it makes a j sound.

And then there are the silent letters!

The following letters can all be silent:

b as in *comb* or *debt*

c as in *scissors*

e as in *make*

g as in *sign* and *gnome*

h as in *what* and *rhinoceros*

k as in *knife*

n as in *autumn*

p as in *psychology*

t as in *listen*

u as in *guess*

w as in *write*

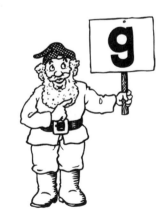

Is it any wonder that children find spelling difficult?

✿ Consonant blends

Consonant blends, as we saw in Chapter 3, are two or more consonant letters, whose sounds blend, with each individual letter retaining its sound.

Consonant blends that appear at the beginning of words are:

br bl cl cr dr fl fr gl gr pl pr sc
scr sk sl sm sn sp spr st str sw tr

Consonant blends that appear at the end of words are:

-ct -ft -ld -lf -lk -lm -lp -lt -mp
-nd -ng -nk -nt -pt -sk -sp -st

✿ Digraphs

Digraphs are two or more letters that join to make one sound. For example: sh as in shop. We first met these in Chapter 3. There are two kinds of digraph, consonant digraphs and vowel digraphs.

Consonant digraphs that appear at the beginning of words are:

ch ph sh th wh

Consonant digraphs that appear at the end of words are:

-ch -ck -sh -tch -th

✿ Vowel digraphs

Vowel digraphs are:

ee ay ai oo ue aw au

In a vowel digraph the sound is made by the first vowel.

Children are often taught how to read these with the saying 'when two vowels go walking the first one does the talking'.

Base words

This is an original word, before any suffixes or prefixes have been added.

For example:

like, help.

Suffixes

A suffix is a letter or group of letters added to the end of a base word to change its use or meaning.

For example:

likely, likeness

There are two types of suffix.

1 Vowel suffix

This is a suffix that begins with a vowel.

For example:

-ed, -ing, -ish

The vowel suffixes are the ones to watch out for, as they often mean you have to change the spelling of the base word before you add them on.

For example: *hope* + *ing* = *hoping*

You have to drop the *e* at the end of *hope* before adding the suffix *ing*.

2 Consonant suffix

This is a suffix that begins with a consonant.

For example:

-less, -ness, -ful, -ly, -ty

These don't usually cause any problems unless you are adding them to a word that ends in *y*.

For example:

happy + *ly* = *happily*

You have to change the *y* to an *i* before adding the suffix.

Prefixes

A prefix is a group of letters added to the beginning of a base word to change its meaning.

For example:

dislike.

Syllables

Words can be split into syllables. This is really important if you find spelling difficult. If you can split a long word into syllables then it will be much easier for you to spell it, as you can concentrate on spelling one syllable at a time.

For example:

helicopter splits into *hel- i- cop- ter*

Think of a syllable like a drum beat in a word. Each syllable has a vowel sound. You can either clap out the syllables or put your hand under your chin and count each time that your chin hits your hand as you say a word.

✿ Types of syllables

There are six types of syllables.

1 Open syllable

An open syllable ends with a vowel. The vowel has a long sound so it says its name.

ta /ble	ā
e /ven	ē
pi /lot	ī
o /pen	ō
mu /sic	ū

2 Closed syllable

A closed syllable ends with a consonant. The consonant at the end closes in on the vowel, stopping it from making its long sound. Therefore, the vowels in closed syllables are short.

tab /let	ă
met /al	ě
win /dow	ĭ
doc /tor	ŏ
up /set	ŭ

3 Vowel team syllable

A vowel team syllable has two vowels next to each other that together say a new sound.

For example:

ai	**train**/ing	says ā
ea	**tea**/bag	says ē
ee	**keep**/er	says ē
ie	un/**tie**	says ī
oo	bath/**room**	says oo
ou	**count**/er	says ow

4 Vowel-consonant-e syllable

A vowel-consonant-e syllable has *e* at the end of a word. The final *e* is silent. These syllables have another vowel in them that make the vowel sound.

For example:

al/ **pine**

in/ **flate**

5 Consonant-controlled syllables

The consonants **r**, **w** and **y** can affect the sound of a vowel. The consonant controls the vowel and changes the way it is pronounced.

For example:

ar	ga**r**/den
or	fo**r**/get
ir	thi**r**st/y
er	m**er**/maid
ur	n**ur**se
ow	sho**w**er
aw	dra**w**
ew	f**ew**
oy	bo**y**
ay	pla**y**
ey	mon**ey**
	th**ey**
uy	b**uy**

6 Regular final syllables

Regular final syllables come at the end of a word.

For example:

sta/**tion**
pic/**ture**
confu/**sion**
ta/**ble**

There are many regular final syllables that end with -le and these are:

-**ble** -**cle** -**ckle** -**dle** -**fle** -**gle** -**kle** -**ple** -**stle** -**tle** -**zle**

So now, we have the basic building blocks for the English language.

It is worth spending a little time becoming familiar with these terms and also practising how to split words into syllables.

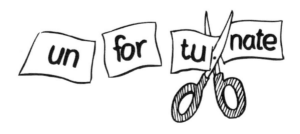

Can you split the following words into syllables? Can you identify what each type of syllable is?

For example:

inspection

This word has three syllables:

in- spec- tion
in = closed syllable
spec = closed syllable
tion = regular final syllable.

By splitting this word you have simplified it from a ten-letter word into a three-syllable (or chunk) word. Much easier to read, spell and remember.

Try these for yourself:
(Answers at the end of this chapter on pages 68–69)

① adventure
② denomination
③ goalkeeper
④ illegal

⑤ photograph
⑥ shoplifter
⑦ understandable
⑧ regulate

Breaking words up into syllables is not the only way to help your child to read and spell. There are many other strategies.

Look for small words within a word

In the word hippopotamus there are the following small words:

hip po pot am us

Identify the prefixes and suffixes

Look at the word unhelpful. Split it into syllables.

un- help- ful

un is a prefix. It is added to the beginning of a base word.

help is the base word. This is the original word before the prefix and suffix were added.

ful is a suffix. It is added to the end of a word.

If you are familiar with spelling prefixes and suffixes then all you have to worry about here is how to spell the word **help.**

There is a list of some of the more common prefixes and suffixes in the resources and information section on pages 105–108.

Say it wrong to spell it right

Pronouncing some words incorrectly can help us to spell them.

For example:

> **Wednesday**. Pronounce this as **Wed - nes- day**
> **people**. Pronounce this as **pe- op- le.**

Use mnemonics and other memory aids

For tricky words, such as **could**, it is useful to use a mnemonic.

> **could:** **C**ats **O**nly **U**pset **L**ittle **D**ogs

Or

> **S**am **A**nd **I** **D**ance

is a good way of remembering the word **said.**

If you are going to use mnemonics with your child, it helps if they can think of the sentences themselves. The sillier the image that they conjure up the better, as this will make it easier for them to remember.

Identify word families

To put it another way, look for common spelling patterns. If your child can recognise common letter strings in words, this will greatly reduce the load on their memory.

For example if they can recognise that **ight** says **īt** (a long i sound followed by **t**) then they will have no problem reading the following words:

> **right, sight, night, fright, might, bright, slight, tonight**
> (etc.)

Furthermore, if you teach them the mnemonic:

> **ight = I G**o **H**ome **T**onight

then they will have no trouble spelling these words either.

A list of common word families is given in the resources and information section on pages 97–104.

Answers to syllable questions on page 66

① adventure	ad	ven	ture		

ad	= closed syllable
ven	= closed syllable
ture	= regular final syllable

② denomination	de	nom	in	a	tion

de	= open syllable
nom	= closed syllable
in	= closed syllable
a	= open syllable
tion	= regular final syllable

③ goalkeeper	goal	keep	er

goal	= vowel team syllable
keep	= vowel team syllable
er	= consonant controlled syllable

④ illegal	il	le	gal

il	= closed syllable
le	= open syllable
gal	= closed syllable

⑤ photograph	pho	to	graph

pho	= open syllable
to	= open syllable
graph	= closed syllable

⑥ **shoplifter**	shop lift er

shop	=	closed syllable
lift	=	closed syllable
er	=	consonant controlled syllable

⑦ **understandable**	un der stand a ble

un	=	closed syllable
der	=	consonant controlled syllable
stand	=	closed syllable
a	=	open syllable
ble	=	regular final syllable

⑧ **regulate**	reg u late

reg	=	closed syllable
u	=	open syllable
late	=	vowel-consonant-e syllable

Don't worry too much if you could not identify the different types of syllable.
The important skill is the ability to split the long words into syllables.

Chapter 7

Games

Overview

Reading and spelling games

Pairs

Link Game

Odd Word Out

Hippopotamus

Happy Families

Spot It

Post It

Silly Syllables

Noughts and Crosses

Writing and grammar games

Word and Picture Card Game

Sentence Pyramid

Consequences

Instant Poem

World of Words

Silly Sentences

Memory games and techniques

Kim's Game

I Went to Market

Alphabet Rainbow

Some memory techniques

There are many useful games and resources that you can buy. I have given details of online games that are readily available in the resources and information section on pages 137–140. However, there are many advantages to making your own games.

- It is cheaper.
- Your child can make them with you. Involving them in this process will make it much more likely that they will want to play the games.
- You can make games specific to your child's actual needs and you can personalise them, using names of friends or pets or objects to which they particularly relate.
- It is fun. No, really, it is...

I have categorised the games into the three following sections:

- Games to improve reading and spelling
- Games to improve writing and grammar
- Games to improve memory.

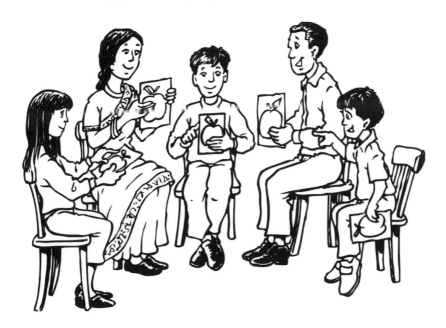

Games to improve reading and spelling

✿ Flashcards

Flashcards are needed in many of the following games. To make the cards you will need:

    A4 card, coloured if possible
    Felt tip pens
    Scissors

Cut the card into 16 rectangles, by folding it in half lengthwise twice and then in half widthwise twice. A guillotine type cutter is useful for this (but not essential).

A photocopiable set of blank cards is supplied on page 88. Alternatively, use blank business card-sized cards, which are available from most office suppliers.

Pairs

This game has countless applications. We will start with the simplest one.

Word Match

Decide on the list of words that you want to work on. Let's say that you are working on the **tch** spelling. Select 12 words and make two sets of cards.

Set 1 and set 2 (both the same)
> **batch, catch, crutch, ditch, fetch, hutch, match, patch, pitch, scratch, switch, witch**

Write these words onto the two sets of 12 cards.

If available, choose a different colour card for set 2 and ask your child to copy the words onto this new set of cards, using a broad felt tip and whatever colour they choose. It can also be helpful to add an illustration at this point. This does not need to be a picture of the word on the card. Picture association is an excellent way of helping children to remember. The more bizarre and silly the association then the more easily they will remember. So, while it is fine for them to draw a picture of a witch on the card that says **witch**, it is just as useful for them to draw a frog in a pointy black hat!

Now place your set of cards, set 1, face down on the table in random order.

Next to these, place your child's set of cards, set 2, face down in random order.

Each player then takes it in turns to select two cards, one from each set. They have to read the word aloud. If the words match then they can keep this pair. If they don't match then they have to replace the cards face down and the next player takes their turn. Play continues until all the words are matched. This game will help your child's reading skills, and also help to improve their memory.

When all the pairs are matched, quickly go over them with your child.

Don't spend too long on this or it could begin to feel like work! You may want to quickly read them again, or ask the child how many of the words they can remember or even ask them to spell or write some of the words.

There are, of course, many different versions of this game:

Word-Word Meaning

For this version, you need one set of cards with the words on and another set with the word meanings. The word has to be matched to its meaning.

For example: **hutch** would pair up with **A home for a rabbit**.

⊙ Word-Sentence Fill

You will need one set of cards with the words written on them and another with a sentence that has that particular word missing.

For example:

witch would pair up with *The .... cast a spell on the prince.*

⊙ Picture-Word

For this version, the word card will pair up with a picture of the word.
This is a great activity to do with a younger child who loves drawing!

⊙ Word-Suffix

There are endless ways of playing this, but you may want to start with a set of cards and a choice of three suffixes.

Set 1

fall, gold, hand, help, jump,
rest, spend, stress, thank, thick

Set 2

en, en, ful, ful, ful, ful, ing, ing, ing, ing

The idea here is to match the word to a suffix that will make a new word.

So *fall* will match with *en* or *ing* but not with *ful*.

⊙ Word-Prefix

This is the same as the previous suffix game but relates to prefixes instead.
So an example of the two sets of cards may be:

Set 1

correct, direct, do, dress, happy, helpful,
place, print, side, use

Set 2

in, in, in, mis, mis, mis, un, un, un, un

⊙ Word-Word Plural

This is useful for words with complicated plurals. For example you may decide to use the following words:

Set 1

baby, cherry, child, fox, knife, leaf,
man, person, wish, woman

Set 2

babies, cherries, children, foxes, knives, leaves, men,
people, wishes, women

Link Game

In this game, each card will link to the next one until all the cards have been used. This is an ideal game for ensuring that your child understands the meaning of more complex words.

How to play
....

Write the words you want to learn onto cards.

Take a card, turn it over and write the meaning for **the next card**.

Continue until the last card, whose meaning clue needs to be written on the back of the first card.

Place all the cards on the table with the clues facing up.

Turn one card over and match it with the correct meaning.

Turn that card over and match it with the correct meaning.

Continue until all the cards have been matched.

Children will enjoy making this game with you and love to make up their own clues as to the meaning of the word.

You can also use this for spelling, by having pictures linking to words. Your child will look at the picture, spell the word and then find it from the cards on the table.

Odd Word Out

This is just like the card game Old Maid. The deck of cards is made up from pairs of the words that you want to learn. One card is removed to create an 'odd word out'. The cards are then dealt between the players and all pairs of words are read aloud and placed in the middle of the table. Players then take it in turns to select a card from another player to try to complete their pair. The loser is the player who has the 'odd word out' card at the end of the game.

Hippopotamus

This is a version of the Odd Word Out game, in which the focus is on syllables. Players have to collect pairs of words with the same number of syllables. There is only one word in the pack with five syllables and that is the word **hippopotamus**. This is a great game to help children to identify syllables in words and can be tailored for any level of ability.

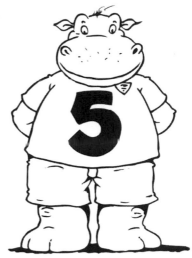

Happy Families

We are all familiar with the card game Happy Families and this is just an adaptation of that. Select the spelling patterns that you are working on. In this example, I will use different ways of spelling the long vowel **a**.

There must be either three or four members of each family.

For example:

train, paid, nail

stay, play, day

cake, same, male

acorn, able, paper

eight, weigh, sleigh

Deal out these cards between the players, who then try to make families of three cards by selecting cards one at a time from each other. When a family of three is made, all of the words must be read out correctly before the family can be placed on the table.

Spot It

Place cards with the words that you are focusing on, one word per card, face up on a table. Use a stopwatch to time your child. Call out a word and your child has to spot the card with that word and grab it. Record how long it takes to spot all the words and try to beat this time when they next play.

Post It

(See page 34.) This is essentially the same as Spot It but uses a post box to put the card into.

Silly Syllables

 You will need:

A Snakes and Ladders board.

A set of cards with pictures on one side and the corresponding word written on the other. These can be any words at all but they need to have different numbers of syllables in them. Animals are useful for this game as they are not too hard to draw and have varying syllable length. For example: **cat** (1), **elephant** (3), **rhinoceros** (4).

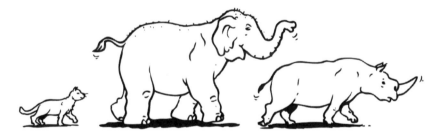

 How to play

Place your counter on the board on the start square. Pick a card and count the syllables in the word. Move that number of places. Go up the ladders and down the snakes as usual. The only difference is that you are counting syllables rather than using dice.

The winner is the first to reach the Finish square.

Noughts and Crosses

back	sack	tick
pick	neck	peck
sock	lock	duck

You will need.

A board of nine squares with one target word written in each square.
A photocopiable blank board for this game is supplied on page 89.

(If you have access to a laminator you could laminate a blank playing board
and then write the target words on with a dry wipe pen. This way, once your
child has mastered the words you can simply wipe them off and write in your
new set of target words.)

Two sets of coloured counters – or a few 1p and 5p coins.

How to play

Player 1 takes a counter or coin and reads one of the words on the board.
If they have read it correctly then they can place their counter over the word.
Once they have covered the word the player will then have to spell the word.

Player 2 now has their turn.

The first player to cover three words, horizontally, vertically or diagonally is
the winner.

This can be extended to larger grids, where your child will have to get four
or five in a row.

Games to improve writing and grammar

 ## Word and Picture Card Game

Make a set of cards with words or pictures of objects, which you can cut out from magazines. Use anything that you can think of! For example:

washing machine, computer, tissues, beef burger, helicopter.

Your child will choose a card without revealing it to you. Then they have to write three sentences to describe the object without actually naming it.

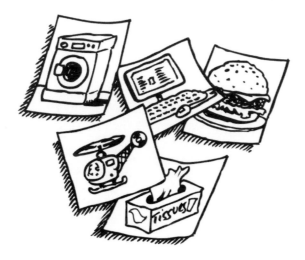

Sentence Pyramid

On a sheet of paper, write the name of an object, for example:

The dog...

Underneath your child has to copy **The dog** and add a word:

The dog ran...

Now it is your turn. It is helpful for you to take a turn at this stage so that you can control the sentence to make sure that it makes sense.

The dog ran quickly...

Continue until you have made a complete sentence.

This activity is also useful for reading and spelling practice. You can make sure that you have included target words when it is your turn to add to the sentence.

Consequences

This is an extension of the Sentence Pyramid game and is universally popular.

Two players can take it in turns to complete the Consequences sheet, folding over their words as they go.

When all the sections have been completed, then the full story can be revealed. Again, the sillier the better.

☉ Consequences template

1 Adjective(s) (a describing word such as **happy**)

2 Name of person or thing

3 Adjective(s)

4 Name of person or thing

5 Where they met

6 What they said

7 Where they went

8 What they did

9 What the consequence was.

Instant Poem

This is a quick way for your child to write poetry. You can make it a nonsense poem if you like or keep it to a specific theme. I have used a seaside theme to illustrate this. A photocopiable blank grid is supplied for you on page 90.

☉ Seaside

Adjective	Noun	Adverb	Verb
impenetrable	castles	proudly	standing
happy	children	quickly	digging
frothing	waves	gently	flowing
sandy	walls	slowly	falling

Your child can either leave their poem as it is or use it as a base for a more complex poem. Once the framework has been completed, your child will find it much easier to edit and improve.

World of Words

Some dyslexic children find it very hard to come up with imaginative vocabulary. They tend to use words like **big**, **good** and **nice**. This activity will help them to expand their vocabulary.

The table below gives an example to help you start. A photocopiable blank table is supplied on page 91. The idea is for your child to come up with as many alternative words as they can for the target words. They can use a thesaurus to help them if they need to.

Then, once the table has been completed, they need to write a sentence or two containing all of the new words.

Target word	1	2	3	4
big	huge	massive	gigantic	colossal
hot				
small				
happy				
dirty				
lovely				
nice				

Therefore, for the word **big** you may end up with something like this:

The colossal giant heaved his huge suitcase into the massive truck. He was going on a gigantic journey around the world.

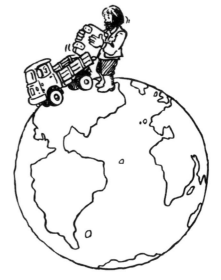

Silly Sentences

This game needs a little more planning but is worth the effort. The idea of the game is similar to Happy Families, but players need to collect the components of a sentence. They will need:

a **noun** / a **verb** / a **preposition** / an **adjective** / and finally another **noun**.

For example:

The dragon / slipped / on a / rickety / bridge.

Once you have the hang of it you can make up your own word banks, but I have given some suggestions here to get you started.

For younger children use different coloured card for each set of words, as this will make it easier for them to construct their sentences in the correct order.

☉ Subject nouns

the queen, a goldfish, my brother, our teacher,
Old King Cole, Humpty Dumpty, the pilot

☉ Verbs

tip-toed, hurtled, screeched, whispered, flick–flacked,
jumped, zoomed

☉ Prepositions

into, on top of, underneath, through, next to, over, around

☉ Adjective phrase

a hairy, the bumpy, a stinky, the enormous, a terrifying,
a spooky, the ugly

☉ Object nouns

bench, sea, swamp, playground, dinosaur, fisherman,
hairdresser

☉ Example sentence:

A goldfish jumped over a stinky dinosaur.

As an added memory exercise, your child can try to remember the sentences that they have made – without looking at the cards.

Games and techniques to improve memory

Helping your child to improve their visual and auditory memory will be one of the most helpful things that you can do for them. It is no good learning how to read and spell dozens of different words if they then can't remember any of them.

The following games are simple to play and require little or no equipment.

Kim's Game

This is a familiar game, but very valuable for improving visual memory.

 How to play

Take a selection of objects, maybe only five or six at first, and lay them out on a table. Ask your child to look at them for one minute and try to remember them. Then with your child's eyes closed remove one of the objects. Can they tell you which item you have removed?

You can increase the number of objects and decrease the time allowed to memorise them according to how good your child's memory is.

In addition, you could cover all the objects and simply ask them to list as many as they can remember.

This activity can also be used to improve auditory memory. In this case, you just give the child a list of items, then repeat the list with one item omitted.

I Went to Market

Many a car journey has been passed playing this game and there are many different versions of it.

The original game involves one person saying:

I went to market and I bought some … carrots.

The next person has to remember the carrots and think of something else.

I went to market and I bought some carrots and some strawberries.

Play continues until the list is so long that no one can remember it correctly.

Other starters are:

I went on holiday and in my bag I packed...

At the seaside I can see...

In the woods I can see...

At school I can see...

I went into space and I took...

This list is only limited by you and your child's imagination.

Alphabet Rainbow

You will need:

A set of wooden or plastic letters.

How to play

Ask your child to set out the letters in alphabetical order in a rainbow shape.

Now select letters at random. Start with three letters and increase the number when your child can remember three letters easily. Say the letter names to your child and then wait for ten seconds before asking your child to find the letters.

You can alter this game and make it more challenging by asking them to find the letters in reverse alphabetical order. This is quite hard to do but will help to develop your child's working memory.

This game will improve auditory memory but can also be used to improve visual memory by writing down the letters on a card for your child to look at. Give your child about five seconds to remember them before taking the card away.

Distraction

You may find that your child is quite good at remembering things for a short time. This is because they have stored the information in their short-term memory. One way to encourage their brains to transfer information into their long-term memory is to give them a list of items to remember then distract them by doing something else for at least 20 seconds. Then go back and see how many items they can still recall. Start slowly, using only three or four items at first.

Memory techniques

You may be familiar with magicians and illusionists who seem to possess an unbelievable talent for memorising items. There are tried and tested methods that they will use to help them to do this. Below, I will outline for you three of these methods that you can use with your child. Try them all and see which one your child prefers.

Before you try these methods give your child ten picture cards. You can draw them yourself (for the artists among us), cut them from a magazine (for those of us with time on our hands) or select them from a standard picture lotto game (for the rest of us).

Place the cards face up in a row in front of your child and give them two minutes to memorise them in order.

Turn the pictures over and make a note of how many they have recalled in the correct order.

Now try the methods on pages 85–86.

Having completed these three techniques, you should find that there is one that your child prefers. I hope you will be astounded at how much more they can remember when they have made a visual association.

Rhyming Method

Write out the numbers 1 to 10. Then ask your child to think of a word that rhymes with each number.

They will probably come up with a list similar to this one:

1 = bun

2 = shoe

3 = tree

4 = door

5 = hive

6 = sticks

7 = heaven

8 = gate

9 = line

10 = hen

Now select a set of ten suitable pictures and lay them out in front of your child.

This time they are going to make a picture association. For instance if the first picture is of an iron then they need to imagine an iron flattening out a jam bun so all the jam is dripping off the ironing board. Encourage your child to make the associations as vivid and unusual as they can.

Continue until all ten pictures have been associated with the 1 = bun 2 = shoe (etc.) sequence.

Now turn the cards over and see if your child can remember them all in the correct order. You will be amazed.

Picture Links

This association technique can also be used by associating the numbers 1–10 with a picture that looks like that number. So now, your child may come up with something resembling the following list.

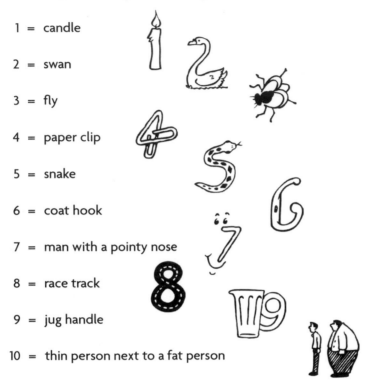

1 = candle

2 = swan

3 = fly

4 = paper clip

5 = snake

6 = coat hook

7 = man with a pointy nose

8 = race track

9 = jug handle

10 = thin person next to a fat person

Then proceed exactly as before. It is important that your child generates their own picture associations for the numbers or they will have difficulty remembering them as well as the list.

Walk around a Room

This time, take your child to a familiar room, for example their bedroom. Then imagine each of the items on your list placed in bizarre and impossible places around the room. Make sure that your child spends a few minutes on this so that they have a good visual image in their mind. Now leave the room and ask your child to recall the items on the list.

Sleep learning

Now, don't panic, this isn't brainwashing your child as they sleep, but it is a technique that is founded on sound psychological research.

Let's assume that the dreaded spelling list has come home in your child's school bag. You will need to spend 10–15 minutes trying to learn these in the usual way. Using the 'look, cover, copy, say, write' method would be a good strategy.

Now leave the spellings and let your child have their tea, watch TV or have a bath, whatever their evening routine is. Then as they go to bed spend a few minutes just quickly going over the spellings again.

Then repeat this first thing in the morning.

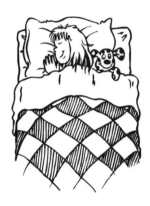

The last thing you think of before you go to sleep and the first thing you think of when you wake up are usually things that your mind is focusing on, even subconsciously. This technique can really help you to remember information that is otherwise easy to forget.

Use this method with caution and only for spellings that they are finding particularly difficult. It wouldn't be something that I would do every night and you will need to judge if it is working for your child, but it is certainly worth a go.

The psychology behind this is the 'little and often' technique. The more often you revisit a piece of information, the more likely you are to be able to store it in your long-term memory. That is why we remember our phone numbers and addresses so easily – we say or write them so frequently.

Pairs Games

© *Help! My Child has Dyslexia* LDA   Permission to photocopy

Noughts and Crosses

Instant Poem

Adjective	Noun	Adverb	Verb

World of Words

Target word	1	2	3	4

Final word

When I first found out that Sam was dyslexic, a friend of mine kindly told me of an article that she had read talking about dyslexia being a 'gift'. I was so angry that I didn't talk to her for many weeks, as I did not see my son's distress and frustration at being unable to read as any sort of gift at all. However, being dyslexic has made Sam develop strategies for learning that he would possibly not have developed otherwise and in many ways has brought us closer together. Over the many years that I have been teaching dyslexic children I have certainly found it true that many are highly creative and have the ability to think 'outside of the box'.

So take heart. Although this is not the road that you would have chosen for your child to travel on, there are ways that you can help and I hope that you and your child will find this book valuable.

And remember, your child is in great company, as the following people are all known to be or have been dyslexic:

Albert Einstein, Walt Disney, Kiera Knightly, Richard Branson, Picasso, Jamie Oliver, Leonardo da Vinci, Winston Churchill, Tom Cruise, John Lennon, Alexander Graham Bell.

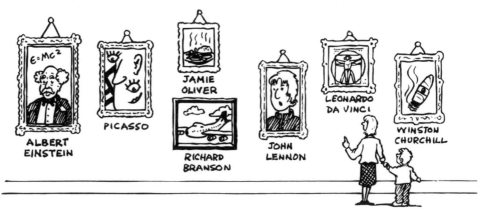

Useful resources and information

Note: You are welcome to photocopy pages from this section for use in your games and activities.

1 The 44 phonemes (sounds) in the English language

The 20 vowel phonemes

short a	a (apple)						
short e	e (egg)	ea (bread)					
short i	i (ink)	y (pyramid)	ui (build)				
short o	o (on)	a (watch)					
short u	u (up)	o (love)	ou (double)				
long a	ai (train)	ay (play)	a-e (cake)	a (able)	eigh (eight)	ei (vein)	ey (grey)
long e	e (even)	ee (sweet)	ea (pea)	ie (shield)	y (baby)	ey (key)	ei (ceiling)
long i	i (ice)	i-e (kite)	ie (tie)	igh (night)	y (try)		
long o	o (open)	o-e (code)	oa (coat)	ow (snow)			
long u	u (unit)	u-e (tune)	ue (due)	eu (Europe)	ew (new)		
long oo	oo (food)	ue (blue)	ou (soup)	ew (chew)	u-e (rule)	oe (shoe)	ui (juice)
short oo	oo (look)						
ou	ou (proud)	ow (crown)					
oi	oi (boil)	oy (toy)					
ar	ar (car)	a (father)					
or	or (port)	aw (dawn)	au (autumn)	ore (store)	oar (oar)	oor (door)	our (pour)
er	er (herb)	ir (bird)	ur (fur)	ear (pearl)			
air	air (pair)	ear (bear)	are (care)				
ear	ear (ear)	eer (cheer)	ere (here)				
schwa ə*	er (sister)	ure (picture)	our (harbour)	ar (collar)	or (doctor)		

* The schwa (ə) sound is the indistinct sound at the end of words such as doctor, sister, baker, picture.

The 24 consonant phonemes

b	b (bed)	bb (rubber)			
c	c (cat)	k (king)	ck (sock)	q (quit)	que (antique)
d	d (dog)	dd (ladder)	ed (watered)		
f	f (fish)	ff (cuff)	ph (photo)	gh (laugh)	
g	g (get)	gg (egg)	gh (ghost)		
h	h (hat)	wh (whole)			
j	j (jam)	g (gentle)	ge (cage)	dge (bridge)	
l	l (leg)	ll (bell)	le (table)		
m	m (men)	mm (hammer)	mb (comb)	mn (column)	
n	n (not)	nn (banner)	kn (knit)	gn (gnat)	
p	p (pin)	pp (slipper)			
r	r (run)	rr (borrow)	wr (write)	rh (rhino)	
s	s (sun)	ss (loss)	ce (face)	c (circle)	sc (science)	ps (psychic)
t	t (tip)	tt (shutter)	ed (picked)	bt (debt)	
v	v (van)	ve (love)			
w	w (wind)	wh (why)	u (quick)		
x	x (fox)				
y	y (yell)				
z	z (zip)	zz (jazz)	ze (craze)	s (dogs)	se (choose)
sh	sh (ship)	ch (chin)	si (fusion)	ti (station)	xi (anxious)
ch	ch (chip)	tch (witch)			
th	th (them)				
ng	ng (ring)				

2 Word families

Use these lists to help you when making up your games cards.

ack	ad	ail	ain	ake	ale	all	am
attack	ad	ail	brain	awake	ale	all	dam
back	bad	fail	chain	bake	bale	ball	dram
black	clad	hail	complain	brake	dale	call	exam
crack	dad	jail	explain	cake	gale	fall	ham
hack	glad	mail	gain	fake	male	gall	jam
lack	had	nail	grain	flake	pale	hall	ram
pack	lad	pail	main	lake	sale	install	Sam
quack	mad	rail	obtain	make	scale	small	scam
rack	pad	sail	pain	quake	stale	squall	slam
sack	sad	snail	plain	rake	tale	stall	spam
snack		tail	rain	sake	whale	tall	swam
stack		wail	Spain	shake		wall	tram
tack			sprain	snake			
track			stain	stake			
			strain	take			
			train	wake			
			vain				

ame	an	ank	ap	ar	ash	at	ate
blame	an	bank	cap	afar	ash	at	abate
came	ban	blank	clap	bar	bash	bat	ate
fame	bran	drank	flap	car	brash	cat	crate
flame	can	frank	gap	far	cash	chat	date
frame	fan	plank	lap	guitar	clash	fat	debate
game	flan	prank	map	jar	crash	flat	fate
lame	man	rank	nap	scar	dash	hat	gate
name	pan	sank	scrap	spar	flash	mat	grate
same	plan	shrank	slap	star	gash	pat	hate
shame	ran	spank	snap	tar	lash	rat	late
tame	scan	tank	strap		mash	sat	mate
	span	thank	tap		rash	slat	plate
	tan	yank	trap		slash	spat	rate
	than		wrap		smash	tat	relate
	van		yap		splash	that	skate
			zap		thrash	vat	state

aw	ay	eat	eel	eep	eet	ell	en
caw	away	beat	eel	beep	beet	bell	amen
claw	bay	cheat	feel	creep	feet	cell	Ben
draw	clay	eat	heel	deep	fleet	dwell	children
flaw	day	feat	kneel	jeep	greet	farewell	den
gnaw	decay	heat	peel	keep	meet	fell	fen
jaw	delay	meat	reel	peep	sheet	sell	gentlemen
law	display	neat	steel	seep	sleet	shell	glen
paw	hay	seat	wheel	sheep	street	smell	hen
raw	jay	treat		sleep	sweet	spell	men
saw	lay	wheat		steep	tweet	swell	open
straw	may			sweep		tell	pen
thaw	pay			weep		well	then
	play					yell	ten
	pray						when
	ray						wren
	relay						
	replay						
	say						
	spray						
	stay						
	stray						
	sway						
	today						
	tray						
	way						

ent	est	ice	ick	ide	ife	ight	ile
bent	best	dice	brick	bride	knife	bright	file
dent	chest	ice	chick	decide	life	delight	mile
event	crest	mice	click	glide	strife	fight	Nile
gent	jest	nice	flick	hide	wife	flight	pile
lent	nest	price	kick	pride		fright	smile
rent	pest	rice	lick	ride		height	stile
scent	quest	slice	nick	side		knight	tile
sent	rest	spice	pick	slide		light	vile
spent	test	splice	quick	stride		might	while
tent	unrest	twice	sick	tide		night	
vent	vest	vice	slick	wide		plight	
went	west		stick			right	
	zest		thick			sight	
			tick			slight	
			trick			tight	
			wick			tonight	

ill	in	ine	ing	ink	ip	it	oat
bill	bin	brine	bring	blink	blip	admit	boat
chill	chin	decline	cling	brink	chip	bit	coat
dill	din	define	fling	drink	dip	fit	float
drill	fin	dine	king	ink	drip	flit	gloat
fill	grin	fine	ping	link	flip	grit	goat
frill	in	line	ring	pink	grip	hit	oat
grill	kin	mine	sing	rink	hip	it	stoat
hill	pin	nine	sling	shrink	lip	kit	throat
ill	shin	pine	spring	sink	nip	knit	
mill	sin	shine	sting	stink	quip	lit	
pill	skin	shrine	string	think	rip	mit	
shrill	spin	spine	swing	wink	ship	pit	
sill	thin	swine	thing		sip	quit	
skill	tin	vine	wing		skip	sit	
spill	twin	wine	wring		slip	slit	
still	win				snip	spit	
swill	within				strip	split	
thrill					tip	twit	
till					trip	wit	
will					whip		
					zip		

ock	og	oil	oke	oo	ood	ood (long oo)	oof (long oo)
block	blog	boil	awoke	boo	good	brood	proof
clock	clog	broil	broke	igloo	hood	food	roof
dock	cog	coil	choke	moo	stood	mood	spoof
flock	dog	foil	joke	shoo	wood		
frock	fog	oil	poke	too			
knock	frog	soil	smoke	woo			
lock	hog	spoil	spoke	zoo			
mock	jog	toil	stoke				
o'clock	log		stroke				
rock	slog		woke				
shock	smog		yoke				
smock							
sock							
stock							

oof	ook	oom	ool	oon	oop	oot (long oo)	oot (short oo)
hoof	book	bloom	cool	balloon	coop	boot	foot
woof	brook	boom	drool	goon	droop	hoot	soot
	cook	broom	fool	loon	hoop	scoot	
	crook	doom	pool	moon	loop	shoot	
	hook	gloom	spool	noon	scoop		
	look	groom	stool	soon	snoop		
	nook	loom	tool	spoon	stoop		
	rook	room		swoon	troop		
	shook	zoom					
	took						

op	ore	orn	ot	ought	ould	ouse	out
chop	bore	adorn	blot	bought	could	douse	about
cop	chore	born	cot	brought	should	grouse	clout
crop	core	corn	dot	fought	would	house	out
drop	more	forlorn	forgot	ought		louse	lout
flop	ore	horn	got	sought		mouse	pout
hop	pore	morn	hot	thought		spouse	scout
lop	score	scorn	jot	wrought			shout
mop	shore	shorn	knot				snout
pop	sore	thorn	lot				spout
prop	store	torn	not				stout
shop	swore	worn	plot				trout
stop	tore		pot				
top	wore		rot				
			shot				
			slot				
			spot				
			tot				
			trot				

ow (rhymes with cow)	ow (rhymes with low)	own	uck	ug	ump	un	unk
bow	bow	brown	cluck	bug	bump	bun	bunk
cow	blow	crown	duck	dug	clump	fun	chunk
how	crow	down	luck	hug	dump	gun	drunk
now	flow	drown	muck	jug	grump	nun	dunk
sow	glow	frown	pluck	lug	hump	pun	funk
vow	grow	gown	stuck	mug	jump	run	hunk
wow	low	nightgown	struck	plug	lump	shun	junk
	mow	town	truck	rug	plump	spun	skunk
	row		tuck	shrug	pump	stun	slunk
	show		yuck	smug	rump	sun	spunk
	slow			snug	slump		sunk
	snow			tug	stump		trunk
	sow				thump		
	stow				trump		
	throw						
	tow						

Regular final syllables

ture	tion	ble	fle	ple	tle	dle	kle
capture	action	bible	raffle	ample	battle	candle	ankle
culture	addition	crumble	baffle	crumple	beetle	cradle	buckle
future	creation	double	shuffle	people	cattle	fondle	crackle
fracture	fraction	horrible	sniffle	sample	kettle	handle	pickle
lecture	fiction	possible	trifle	simple	little	needle	sprinkle
mixture	motion	table	waffle	staple	title		tickle
nature	nation	treble					twinkle
picture	relation						
posture	portion						
structure	station						
	subtraction						

cle	gle	zle	stle	age	cian	sion	ous
article	angle	dazzle	bristle	bandage	electrician	confusion	anxious
circle	bangle	drizzle	bustle	cabbage	magician	decision	dangerous
cycle	giggle	nozzle	castle	cottage	optician	division	enormous
miracle	juggle	puzzle	jostle	damage	politician	illusion	famous
obstacle	jungle		nestle	garage	musician	invasion	furious
particle	rectangle		thistle	image		mansion	glorious
spectacle	single		whistle	luggage		revision	nervous
treacle	snuggle		wrestle	message		television	serious
uncle	struggle			package			spacious
vehicle	tangle			postage			various
	triangle			shortage			
				village			

3 Prefixes and suffixes

Prefixes

Prefix	Meaning	Example
ab	away from	abnormal
aero	to do with air	aeroplane
anti	against	antifreeze
auto	by yourself	autobiography
bi	two	bicycle
bio	life	biology
centi	hundred	centimetre
circum	around	circumference
co	jointly	co-operate
contra	against	contradict
cross	across/from two types	crossbar/crossbreed
de	removing/down	defrost/descend
deci	one-tenth	decimal
dis	the reverse of	dishonest
equi	equally	equilateral
ex	out	extract
extra	beyond	extraordinary
fore	in front of	forecast
homo	same	homophone

hydro	**water**	hydrofoil
il	**not**	illegal
im	**not**	immature
in	**not**	incorrect
inter	**between**	interact
ir	**not**	irregular
kilo	**thousand**	kilogram
mal	**bad**	malnutrition
mega	**large**	megaphone
micro	**very small**	microscope
milli	**one thousandth**	millilitre
mini	**very small**	minibus
mis	**badly**	misfit
mono	one	monotone
multi	many	multicultural
non	not	nonfiction
octo	eight	octopus
out	away/separate/more than	outcast/outhouse/outdo
over	too much	overcrowd
photo	light	photograph
poly	many	polygon
post	after	postpone
pre	before	prefix
re	again	rewind
semi	half	semicircle
sub	under	subway
super	bigger	supermarket
tele	far	television

trans	across	transport
tri	three	triangle
un	not/reverse	uncertain/unwind
uni	one	uniform

Suffixes

Vowel suffixes

Suffix	Meaning/use	Example
able	forms an adjective	readable
ary	to do with	secondary
ate	forms an adjective	passionate
ed	forms a past tense	painted
er	comparative/a person who does	faster/swimmer
est	forms a superlative	fastest
ible	forms an adjective	sensible
ic	forms an adjective	chaotic
ician	person skilled in something	magician
ing	shows action of a verb	hearing
ish	of a certain nature/rather	foolish/yellowish
y (treated as a vowel)	to do with/like	sticky/messy

Consonant suffixes

Suffix	Meaning/use	Example
ful	full of	truthful
gram	something written	diagram
graph	something recorded in some way	photograph
hood	condition or quality	childhood
less	without	colourless
ly	makes adverbs from adjectives	quickly
ness	makes nouns from adjectives	sadness
ship	condition or skill	friendship/seamanship
ward	shows direction	forward
wise	in this manner or direction	clockwise

4 Homophones

This is a list of words that sound the same but are spelt differently, with examples showing the correct spelling for each word.

aisle/isle/I'll

The bride walked up the aisle.
I went to visit the Isle of Wight.
I'll be coming home tomorrow.

allowed/aloud

Children are not allowed to use the spa.
Read aloud so that I can hear you.

alter/altar

We had to alter the timetable.
The vicar was standing in front of the altar.

ate/eight

I ate all my lunch.
Today I am eight years old.

aural/oral

His aural skills were poor as he was a bit deaf.
The dentist talked about good oral hygiene.

band/banned

My brother plays guitar in a rock band.
The angry man was banned from the meeting.

bare/bear

There was no food in the house so the cupboard was bare.
My favourite toy is my teddy bear.

beach/beech

I love sunbathing on the beach.
There was a huge beech tree in the garden.

blew/blue

She blew the balloon up until it burst.
The girl had a blue dress.

board/bored

The teacher wrote the lesson on the board.
The boy was bored as he had nothing to do.

brake/break

The car had to brake suddenly when it went round a sharp bend.
I had a biscuit during my coffee break.

buy/by/bye

I would like to buy a new car this year.

I have to walk by the cinema on my way to school.

It is time to go so 'Bye Bye'.

cue/queue

The actor missed his cue in the second act.

There was a long queue at the bus stop.

dear/deer

My mother is so dear to me.

The deer fled as he saw the headlights.

fair/fare

It is not fair that I can't go to the party.

The bus fare was £2.50.

feat/feet

Climbing the mountain alone was an amazing feat.

The teenage boy had smelly feet.

flour/flower

Use strong flour when baking bread.

The flower garden was beautiful.

for/four

I went for a walk.

I have four books to read.

grate/great

Grate some cheese for me please.

This holiday is great fun.

groan/grown

The joke was so bad it made the audience groan.

My school blazer won't fit because I have grown so much.

hair/hare

My hair was blonde but I have dyed it black.

The hare raced across the field into its burrow.

heal/heel

The doctor was able to heal my leg.

My new shoes were rubbing the heel of my foot.

hear/here

I can't hear you, can you speak a bit louder?

Come over here, right away!

heard/herd

I heard you the first time. You don't need to say it again.

A herd of cows were grazing in the field.

hole/whole

The girl tore a hole in her dress.

The greedy boy ate the whole cake.

hour/our

The exam lasted for one hour.

It is our turn to go out to play.

its/it's

The dog lost its bone.

It's sunny today.

knew/new

I knew you were coming so I baked
 a cake.
Do you like my new dress?

knight/night

The knight wore shining armour.
It gets dark at night.

leak/leek

The water pipe sprung a leak.
I like to eat leeks with cheese sauce.

made/maid

I made a chocolate cake.
The maid had not cleaned the
 room yet.

meat/meet

I am a vegetarian so I don't eat
 meat.
I was going to meet my friend at
 the cinema.

one/won

I have one daughter.
I won the tennis match.

pain/pane

I had a pain in my neck.
The window pane was broken.

pair/pear

I have a pair of pink socks.
My favourite fruit is pear.

pause/paws

Pause the video so I can make a
 cup of tea.
The cat had muddy paws.

peace/piece

The children were asleep so I had
 some peace at last.
I will have another piece of cake,
 please.

pray/prey

I go to church to pray.
The bird of prey ate the mouse.

rain/reign/rein

It is sure to rain on our day out.
The queen has had a long reign on
 the throne.
The rider pulled on the horse's rein.

read/red

I have read all the books in my
 room.
My new dress was red.

right/write

That spelling is not right.
Can you write me a letter please?

road/rode/rowed

The road was long and twisty.
I rode my bike to the shops.
We rowed the boat across the
 Channel.

sail/sale

The ship put its sail up.
The dress shop had a half price sale.

scent/sent

The scent of the rose was
 intoxicating.
I sent a letter to my cousin in
 America.

sea/see

The sea was too cold to swim in.
I can see the field from my room.

sew/so/sow

I need to sew the hem on my dress.
I have a cold so I am staying in bed.
The farmer had to sow the seed.

stair/stare

The stair creaked as I entered the
    haunted house.
It is rude to stare at someone.

stationary/stationery

The road accident caused the traffic
    to be stationary for miles.
I bought my pen at the new
    stationery shop.

steal/steel

He intended to steal the diamonds.
The cutlery was made from stainless
    steel.

tail/tale

The dog wagged his tail.
The teacher told the boy not to
    tell tales.

threw/through

He threw the ball across the gym.
I walked through the crowd to
    reach the exit.

waist/waste

The skirt was too tight around
    my waist.
Throwing food away is a waste.

wait/weight

I had to wait 15 minutes for the bus.
The beef joint was 2 kilograms in
    weight.

way/weigh

I'm lost. I don't know the way!
How much do you weigh?

wear/where

I shall wear my new shoes tonight.
Where are you going?

weak/week

The old man was too weak to walk
    up the steps.
There are seven days in a week.

which/witch

Which way shall we go?
The witch cast a spell on me.

wood/would

The table was made from oak wood.
I would like to go home now please.

5 The 21 spelling rules and exceptions

Why does the English language have so many words that are difficult to spell?

Well, at the risk of you closing this book and heading for the park instead, it is because there are 150 different ways to spell the 44 sounds in the English language!

These 44 sounds are listed on pages 95–96 with examples of each sound.

Consequently, we have:

- Words that sound the same but are spelt differently, for example *sea* and *see* or *sight* and *site*. These are called homophones and a list of common homophones is given on pages 109–112.
- Words that have letters in them that seem to serve no purpose at all, for example *through* and *antique*.
- Words that contain silent letters, for example *write* and *autumn*.

There are many spelling rules and they can be helpful in giving children something concrete to cling on to in the crazy world of English spelling. However, nothing is ever that simple and you will need to watch out for the exceptions to the rules.

Some children find spelling rules very useful, as the rules give them a reason for why a word is spelt a certain way. However, your child will not be able to remember them all. They should use this section as a reference, so that they can check their own spellings.

1 q is always followed by u

To remember this say:

> q and u stick together like glue.

The sound that qu makes is kw

There are exceptions in words such as *Iraq*.

2 Very few English words end in *i*

Generally English words use **y** for the *i* sound at the end of a word.

There are exceptions, such as **taxi**, which was originally a shortened form of **taxicab**, and **spaghetti**, which was derived from Italian.

3 The *x* and *s* rule

The letter **s** never follows **x** but **c** often does and can be soft or hard.

For example: *except, excite, excellent, exclude, exclaim*

4 Soft and hard sounds

✿ The *k* sound

To decide whether to use **k** or **c**, then you need to look at the vowel that comes after the **k** sound.

Use **k** if the vowel afterwards is **e**, **i** or **y**.
For example: *kettle, king*

The same rule applies to **sk** words.
For example: *sketch, skin, sky*

Use **c** if the vowel afterwards is **a o** or **u**.
For example: *cat, cot, cup*

The same rule applies to **sc** words.
For example: *scab, scotch, scarf*

✿ Soft *c*

If **c** is followed by **e**, **i** or **y** then it will make the soft sound **s**.
For example: *centre, city, cycle*

✿ Soft *g*

A similar rule applies to the **g** sound.

When **g** is followed by **i**, **y** or **e** it usually makes the soft sound **j**.
For example: *gin, gyroscope, gentle*

There are some exceptions to this in words such as:

gear, gelding, get, geyser, giddy, gift, giggle, gild, gimmick, gird, girder, girdle, girl, girth, give, gizzard, gynaecology

5 Silent e

Your child may have learnt about 'magic e' or 'silent e' at school. This is because e often appears at the end of a word but makes no sound.

There are five different uses for e at the end of a word.

✿ Use 1

The e is used to make a short vowel sound into a long vowel sound. For example the word mad has a short ă sound in the middle, but when we add e at the end it says made and the a in the middle now has a long ā sound.

✿ Use 2

The e is used to save us from ending a word in v or u. Neither of these letters is used to end words in English.
For example: love, true

✿ Use 3

The e is used to make a c or g soft.
For example: police, advantage

✿ Use 4

The e is used to stop us having a syllable without a vowel.
For example: peo/ple, dan/gle

✿ Use 5

The e is used to stop a word that is not plural from ending in s.
For example: purse, course

6 The sound er

There are five different sounds for the spelling er. These are er, ur, ir, or and ear and they are used in this order of frequency.

✿ er

er is the most common spelling, so use this if you are in doubt.

Use er for most words showing what someone is doing.
For example: boxer, shopper, singer

✿ ir

Use ir for girl-related words.
For example: girl, skirt, flirt, bird

Also use ir for the numbers: first, third, thirteen and thirty.

✿ ur

Use **ur** for words to do with hurting.

For example:

> surgeon, nurse, hurt, burn

7 Suffixes and prefixes

✿ Suffixes

A suffix is a letter or group of letters added to the end of a base word to change its use or meaning. There are four rules about suffixes.

1 The just add rule

Normally the suffix is just added onto the end of the word.

For example: **help + ing = helping**

However, there are some groups of words that you have to watch out for, namely:

2 The 1-1-1 rule

This is also sometimes called 'the doubling rule'.

It applies to words that have:

> 1 syllable
> 1 short vowel
> and
> 1 consonant at the end.

Happily there is no problem if the suffix that you are adding starts with a consonant, such as *ful* or *less*:

> **help + ful = helpful**

But if the suffix starts with a vowel, then you must double the final consonant of the word before you add the suffix:

> **stop+ ing = stopping**

Note: For these purposes y is treated as a vowel suffix because it makes a vowel sound:

> **sun+ y = sunny**

We don't double **w** or **x** as these letters are never doubled.

> So, **tax** + **ing** = **taxing** (not **taxxing**)
> And **claw** + **ed** – **clawed** (not **clawwed**)

3 The drop e rule

This applies to words that end with a silent **e**.

Again, the rule only applies if you are adding a suffix that begins with
a vowel.

> So, **hope** + **ing** = **hoping**
> But, **hope** + **ful** = **hopeful**

EXCEPTIONS

You need to keep the **e** if you have a soft **g** or a soft **c** word. For example:
outrageous and **noticeable**, as it is the **e** that keeps the **g** and the **c** soft.

However, don't keep the **e** with these awkward words:

> **argument, awful, duly, ninth, truly,**
> **whilst, wisdom, wholly**

4 The change y rule

This rule refers to words that end in **y**.
The key here is to look at the letter that comes before the **y**.

If there is a vowel before the **y** then just add the suffix (even if it begins
with a vowel):

> **play** + **ful** = **playful**
> **play** + **ing** = **playing**

If there is a consonant before the **y** then you change the **y** to an **i**:

> **tidy** + **er** = **tidier**

EXCEPTIONS

If you are adding **ing** then you never change the **y** to an **i** or you
would end up with **ii**.

In addition, the following words don't follow the rule:

> **daily, laid, paid, said, shyly, shyness, dryness**

✿ Prefixes

Sometimes the prefix changes to become more like the base word. The most common prefixes are *ad*, *com*, *in*, *is*, *sub*.

When one of these prefixes is added to a word that starts with one of these letters:

f, s, r, n, p, g, l, t, c

then it changes and becomes a 'changed prefix'.

For example:

ad + firm = affirm
ad + tract = attract
in + legal= illegal
in + regular = irregular
in + mature = immature
com + lapse = collapse
dis + fuse = diffuse
sub + ply = supply
sub + render = surrender

This mnemonic can help you to remember the letters that will cause a prefix to change:

Fiona Says Really Nice People Give Loads To Charity.

Other prefixes can also change:

ex+ fect = effect
ob+ fer = offer

8 'i before e, except after c'

'*i* before *e*, except after *c*, unless it says *a* as in *neighbour* and *weigh*'.

This tells us to spell *field* with the *i* before the *e* but to spell *ceiling* with the *e* before the *i*.

EXCEPTIONS

The exceptions to this rule are the words:

reign, rein, veil, vein, height, eight, weight, heir, seize, weird

9 The l rule

a) When a small word that ends with ll, for example all, is joined to another word, ways, then you drop one l.

This applies whether the word is added at the beginning or the end of the first word.

> all + ways = always
>
> un + till = until

Other examples are:

> almost, altogether, already, fulfil, although, almighty, fulsome, helpful

b) Till and full as single words have two ls but if they are used as suffixes then only one l is used.

10 Sticky i

i sometimes 'sticks' to other letters. When this happens it makes a sh sound.

For example:

> ti makes tion   fraction
>
> ssi makes ssion   mission
>
> ci makes cian   magician
>
> si makes sion   fusion
>
> xi makes xious   anxious

There are only two commonly used words in English that actually have sh making this sh sound and these are the words fashion and cushion.

 tion

tion is the most common of the sticky i words. Always use this spelling pattern if you are not sure which one to use.

Use tion after a long vowel, for example creation, and after a consonant, for example: function.

✿ ssion

ssion is the least common spelling pattern and is used after a short vowel. For example:

> mission

✿ cian

cian is easy to remember as it is only used for people's jobs.

For example: *magician, electrician, optician*

11 Flossy rule

We call this the flossy rule because it applies to words ending in *f l* and *s*. It also applies to *z* and *k*.

The rule states that for one-syllable words with a short vowel sound you need to double the consonant at the end.

For example:

> *cliff, fluff, hill, smell, cross, fuss, jazz, sock, pick*
> (note that you use *ck* not *cc* or *kk*)

EXCEPTIONS

Of course there are exceptions to this rule. These exceptions have a long vowel sound that should really be short.

For example: *kind, post, find, pint, cold*

If you look at the word *pint* it should sound the same as *mint*.

The word *wind* can be long as in *wind up the clock* or short as in *the wind blew my hat off*.

12 Middle or end choices

Some words have sounds that are spelt differently depending on whether they are in the middle or end of the word.

✿ *oa* or *ow*?

Use *oa* at the beginning or in the middle of a word.

For example: *oath, coat*

Use ow at the end of a word.

For example: *snow, follow*

✿ oi or oy?

Use **oi** at the beginning or in the middle of a word.
For example: *oil, coin*

Use **oy** at the end of a word.
For example: *boy, employ*

EXCEPTION
  oyster.

✿ au or aw?

Use **au** at the beginning or in the middle of a word.
For example: *autumn, sauce*

Use **aw** at the end of a word.
For example: *straw, claw*

We also use **aw** before a single **n** or **l**.
For example: *yawn, crawl.*

EXCEPTIONS
  Paul, haul, awful, awkward, hawk, awesome

✿ igh or y?

Use **igh** in the middle of a word.
For example: *sight, right*

Use **y** at the end of a word.
For example: *try, cry*

EXCEPTIONS
These three words have the **igh** spelling at the end:
  sigh, high, thigh

✿ ai or ay?

Use **ai** at the beginning or in the middle of a word.
For example: *aim, sail*

Use **ay** at the end of a word or before a suffix.
For example: *say, saying*

13 Long or short vowel choices

Some spelling choices are determined by whether the vowel sound in the word is long or short.

✿ **ch** or **tch**?

If the vowel is short use **tch**.
For example: *catch, witch, hutch*

If the vowel is long use **ch**.
For example: *reach, beech*

We also use **ch** after a consonant.
For example: *bench, pinch*

EXCEPTIONS
    such, much, rich, which

✿ **dge** or **ge**?

Use **ge** after a long vowel.
For example: *cage, huge, page*

Use **dge** after a short vowel.
For example: *bridge, hedge, fudge*

14 The **ul** sound

-*le*, -*al*, and -*el* all make the same sound – *ul*.

✿ -*le*

le is the most common spelling and is used for words ending in -*ible* and -*able*. However, it is not used after the following letters:

    m, n, r, v, w, u, s

You can remember these letters by using the mnemonic:

    Most **N**uns **R**un **V**ery **W**ell **U**sually **S**aturdays

✿ -*al*

al is used for adjectives.
For example: *final, legal, vital*

✿ -el

el is used for nouns.

For example: *towel, vowel, channel*

There are some nouns that can also be adjectives.

For example: *manual, capital, criminal, individual, intellectual, signal, terminal*

Also, there are some nouns that end in **al**, namely:

  animal, coral, funeral, hospital, jackal, metal, mineral, pedal, sandal

15 o as u

In some words **o** makes a **u** sound, for example in words such as **love**.

Often **o** says **u** before the letters **v, th, n, m**. This is because you can't have **u** and **v** next to each other as they look like the letter **w**. Therefore, you need to use **o** but it will sound like **u**.

16 w, wh and qu

w, wh and **qu** make an **a** say **o**.
For example: *wash, what, wallet, want, squash, quads*

w makes **or** say **er**.
For example: *worm, word, work, world*

w and **qu** make **ar** say **or**.
For example: *war, warm, warn, quarter*

17 Syllable-controlled spellings

Some words use a different spelling pattern or sound depending on whether they have one, or more than one, syllable.

✿ ick or ic?

For one-syllable words use ick.

For example: sick, thick, brick

For words of two or more syllables, use ic.

For example: fantastic, basic, electric

✿ age

For one-syllable words age has a long ā sound.

For example: cage, rage, sage

For two-syllable words age has a short ĭ sound.

For example: cabbage, postage, village

18 ch as k and sh

The English language has been influenced by other languages, such as French, German, Greek and Latin. This is the reason why some of our spellings seem so strange.

We usually use ch for words like chips and bench. However, words that have come from Greek make ch say k.

For example: school, Christmas

Words with French origin make a ch say sh.
For example: chef, chauffeur

19 a before s and th

There is no r before the letters s and th. It is regional variations in dialect that can make the word sound as if there is an r.

For example: bath, pass

20 Ugly green hairy words

There really seems to be no rhyme or reason to these words and they are notoriously difficult to spell. I teach them by calling them Ugly Green Hairy (UGH) words.

They have eight different sounds.

or	o	u	uff
ought, bought, brought, thought, fought, sought, nought, caught, naughty, taught, daughter, slaughter	dough though although doughnut	thorough borough thoroughly	rough tough enough
off	ow	oo	arf
cough trough	plough bough drought	through	laugh laughter

21 Plurals

There are six different rules that you need to remember when spelling plurals.

✿ Just add s

This is the most common way of making a word plural.

For example:

> book – books
> table – tables
> window – windows

✿ Just add es

You will need to add es if the word already has a hissing s sound at the end.

For example:

> bus – buses
> catch – catches
> fox – foxes
> wish – wishes

This is so that you can hear the difference between the single and plural form.

✿ Words ending in y

For these words you need to look at the letter that comes before the y. If there is a vowel before the y then you just add s.

For example:
> toy – toys
> monkey – monkeys

If there is a consonant before the y then you must change the y to an i and add es.

For example:
> baby – babies
> fairy – fairies

✿ Words ending in o

Typically you will just need to add s.

For example:
> piano – pianos   photo – photos
> studio – studios   video – videos

However, there are some exceptions:
> domino – dominoes   mosquito – mosquitoes
> echo – echoes   potato – potatoes
> hero – heroes   tomato – tomatoes

✿ Words ending in -f or -fe

Generally you just add s to these words.

For example:
> chief – chiefs
> giraffe – giraffes
> cliff – cliffs
> roof – roofs

There are some exceptions, where you will need to change the f to ves. For example:
> knife – knives   half – halves
> life – lives   leaf – leaves
> wife – wives   thief – thieves
> self – selves   loaf – loaves
> shelf – shelves   wolf – wolves
> calf – calves

Some words can be spelt either way.
For example:

> *hoofs* or *hooves*
> *scarfs* or *scarves*

✿ Irregular words

Some words are the same in the singular and plural form.
For example:

> *sheep*
> *deer*
> *fish*

Some words change completely.
For example:

> *man – men*   *goose – geese*
> *woman – women*   *mouse – mice*
> *child – children*   *die – dice*
> *foot – feet*

6 Common spelling confusions

I have listed these in alphabetical order.

Advice or **advise**?

Advice is a noun.
You should listen to my **advice.**

Advise is a verb.
Please **advise** me what to do.

Affect or **effect**?

Affect is a verb.
Eating too much will **affect** your weight.

Effect is a noun.
The **effect** of the diet was immediate.

Allowed or **aloud**?

Allowed:
You are not **allowed** to smoke in a restaurant.

Aloud:
She read her story **aloud** to the class.

All together or **altogether**?

All together:
The children went **all together** on the school trip.

Altogether:
This trip was **altogether** different from the last one.

Apostrophes

Apostrophes have two uses.

1 To show when some letters are missing. These are called contractions.

For example: can't, I've, we'll, won't

2 To show possession. In this case the apostrophe is used to show when something belongs to someone. The trick here is to decide who owns the object.

For example: The toy of the child

The child is the owner so we write:

The child's toy

If there is more than one owner then you only need to put an apostrophe after the **s** if there is already one there.

For example: The sandpit of the boys

The boys are the owners so we write:

The boys' sandpit

Aural or oral?

Aural is to do with hearing.
Oral is to do with speaking.

Bought or brought?

Bought
This refers to buying things.
I bought a new dress today.

Brought
This refers to bringing something with you.
I brought cheese and pineapple on sticks to the party.

-cal or -cle word ending?

cle is the ending for nouns.
For example: particle, uncle

cal is the ending for adjectives.
For example: practical, comical

-ed or **-t** word ending?

Some words can be spelled (or spelt!) in two ways. You can use either *ed* at the end or *t*:

burned	burnt	smelled	smelt
dreamed	dreamt	spelled	spelt
kneeled	knelt	spilled	spilt
leaned	leant	spoiled	spoilt
leaped	leapt		

Its or it's?

Its means belonging to it.
The dog wagged **its** muddy tail on the white sofa.

It's is short for *it is*.
It's raining cats and dogs.

Licence or license?

Licence is a noun:
The lorry driver left his driving **licence** in the cafe.

License is a verb:
The landlord of the pub was **licensed** to sell alcohol.

Practice or practise?

Practice is a noun:
It is time to do your piano **practice**.

Practise is a verb:
Please go and **practise** your piano pieces.

There, their and they're?

There
There is a place word and also part of the verb 'to be'.
Put your coat over **there**.
There are fairies at the bottom of my garden.

Their
Their is used for belonging.
The children left **their** homework at school.

They're
They're is short for **they are**.
They're looking forward to a holiday.

To, too or two?

To
To can be used next to a verb:
Would you like to dance?

To is also used in sentences such as this:
Can you give this £50 note to your brother?
How do you get to Wales in a car?

Too
Too can mean 'more than enough':
It is too hot in this car

And too can also mean 'also':
Can I come to the cinema too?

Two
Two is the correct spelling for the number 2:
There are two clowns sitting in the back of my car.

How do you get two whales in a car?

Or putting all three together:
Can the two whales go to Wales too?

Who's or whose?

Who's is short for who is?
Who's making all that noise?

Whose is a question word. It is used to ask questions about who something belongs to.
Whose house is this?

7 Words that are often spelt wrong

Here is a list of the correct spellings of words that are commonly spelt wrong.

A
accidentally
accommodate
apparent
argument

B
because
beautiful

C
calendar
cemetery
changeable
committed
conscience
conscientious

D
definite
discipline

E
embarrass
exhilarate
exceed
existence

F
fiery
foreign

G
gauge
grateful (not **great**)
guarantee

H
harass
height
humorous

I
ignorance
immediate
independent
indispensable
intelligence

J
jewellery

K
knowledge

L
leisure
liaison
library
lightning

M
maintenance
miniature
misspell

N
neighbour
noticeable

O
occasionally
occurrence

P
personnel
playwright
possession
precede
privilege (two [i]s + two [e]s in that order)
pronunciation

Q
queue

R
restaurant
rhyme
rhythm

S
schedule
separate

T
twelfth

U
until

V
vein/vain
(vein = carries blood, vain = loving the way you look)
vacuum

W X Y Z
weird

8 Books for reluctant readers

Books for children aged 5-9

The Cat in the Hat by Dr. Seuss, HarperCollins

> My children adored Dr Seuss books and found them easy to read and memorise. They use phonics and rhyme in a fun way and I highly recommend any of them.

Candyfloss by Jacqueline Wilson and Nick Sharratt, Corgi

> Jacqueline Wilson is a very popular author. She certainly has her finger on the pulse of today's children.

Horrid Henry series by Francesca Simon and Tony Ross, Orion

> Horrid Henry is an excellent character and children love to read of all the terrible things that he gets up to. The chapters are short, easy to cope with and well illustrated.

Slam by Nick Hornby, Penguin

> This book is a good coming-of-age novel, especially for boys. An excellent story with some hilarious moments.

Percy Jackson and the Last Olympian by Rick Riordan, Puffin

> This is an adventure book series whose main character is dyslexic and a superhero. The first book, *The Lightning Thief,* has been made into a film, making the book more accessible to dyslexic readers.

The Bad Beginning by Lemony Snicket, Egmont

> I don't often enjoy reading children's fiction as much as adult fiction, but this series, called *A Series of Unfortunate Events*, is exceptional. It is both dark and funny and a tiny bit scary. Perfect for captivating children's imaginations and for reading together with your child.

Books for children aged 9–12 with a reading age of between 6 and 8 years

To the Extreme by David Gatward, Barrington Stoke

> This is an action-packed, gripping non-fiction book, perfect for reluctant readers who love facts.

The Uniform by Tommy Donbavand, Barrington Stoke

> This is a horror story that tackles the themes of bullying and being accepted. It is an excellent book for the struggling reader.

The Sticky Witch by Hilary McKay, Barrington Stoke

> This hilarious book will have your child laughing out loud. It features Tom, Ellie and their cat, who are sent to stay with their loathed Aunt, the sticky witch.

The Five Lords of Pain: Book 2 The Lord of the Void by James Lovegrove, Barrington Stoke

> Unless warrior Tom can fight and beat all the five demons of the Lords of Pain in a series of duels then the whole world will cease to exist as he knows it.

The Dying Photo by Alan Gibbons, Barrington Stoke

> A gripping ghost story based on a blurb by a Year 6 boy from a Liverpool primary school who won a city-wide competition. A real page-turner that's an excellent story for reluctant readers.

The Hat Trick by Terry Deary, Barrington Stoke

> Terry Deary, one of the most successful and readable writers for children, has once again delivered an excellent short read.

Dino-Hunter by Simon Chapman, Barrington Stoke

> Step back in time to a thrilling adventure in a world where dinosaurs exist and there is deadly danger at every turn.

Hostage by Malorie Blackman, Barrington Stoke

> Malorie Blackman is one of the country's best authors and this short book is unputdownable. The main character, Angela, has been kidnapped. She's blindfolded and alone and fears for her life.

Zombie! by Tommy Donbavand, Barrington Stoke

> Mayhem follows when Jake discovers a party-loving zombie.

Fire Mask by Franzeska G. Ewart, Barrington Stoke

> Josh and a long-standing best friend are now sworn enemies and when the ex-best friend plays a nasty trick on him he swears revenge.

Living with Vampires by Jeremy Strong, Barrington Stoke

> Family problems of an unusual kind make life complicated for Kevin. With vampires for parents, he does his best to control them but things can't help getting out of hand.

Books for children aged 12+

Cliff Edge by Jane A.C. West, Barrington Stoke

> This is a cliffhanger adventure featuring a boy who has to climb unaided to save his friends.

The Number 7 Shirt by Alan Gibbons, Barrington Stoke

> This is an action-packed story involving a boy who dreams of being a football pro.

Icefall by John Townsend, Barrington Stoke

> When Barney is woken in the night by voices outside his room in the ski resort, he knows something suspicious is going on.

Twisting the Truth by Judy Waite, Barrington Stoke

> When Elsa's friend goes missing from school someone is arrested who may be innocent and it's up to Elsa to find out who really abducted her.

Crazy Creatures by Gill Arbuthnott, Barrington Stoke

> A true story that's stranger than fiction, involving a bird that fights by being sick on you, a frog that can kill 1,500 people and many more fabulous facts.

Diary of an (Un)teenager by Pete Johnson, Barrington Stoke

> Spencer is determined that he'll stay exactly as he is when he turns 13. As he tells his diary, he wants nothing to do with the clothes, kit and attitudes that other teenagers adopt.

Reading schemes/series

Wolf Hill series, Oxford University Press

> This is a series written for reluctant readers with an interest age of 7–11 and a reading age of 6–8.

Trackers series, Crick Software/Oxford University Press

> The series is based on the outstanding fiction books from Oxford's *Trackers* structured reading series. For children aged 7+ who have a reading age of 5+.

Wellington Square, Nelson Thornes

> Aimed at 7–11 year olds, this is a very popular reading scheme.

Five / Ten Minute Thrillers, LDA

> These are excellent high interest, low reading age books with gripping storylines. Interest level 9+ and 11+, reading level 8.

9 Useful websites

Information and advice

British Dyslexia Association

www.bdadyslexia.org.uk

> This is a national organisation, offering a wide range of information for parents, dyslexic adults and teachers. It has some particularly useful advice on where and how to have your child assessed and also on how to deal with schools.

Being Dyslexic

www.beingdyslexic.co.uk

> Being Dyslexic is a website for anyone with dyslexia, or anyone interested in finding out about dyslexia.

PATOSS

(Professional Association of Teachers of Students with Specific Learning Difficulties)
www.patoss-dyslexia.org

> This website provides contact details of specialist teachers.

Dyslexia Action

www.dyslexiaaction.org.uk

> This website provides information about dyslexia services, dyslexia associated training, teaching and publication details.

National Grid for Learning

www.inclusion.ngfl.gov.uk

> The National Grid for Learning Inclusion site.

The Literacy Trust

www.literacytrust.org.uk

>Provides information, links and resources on literacy.
>An interesting and user-friendly site.

Dyslexia Help

www.dyslexichelp.org

>This site is aimed at parents of dyslexic children and is packed with resources and information.

World of Dyslexia

www.dyslexia-parent.com/world_of_dyslexia.html

>A very useful site for parents and teachers alike.

Dyslexia Information

www.dyslexia-information.com

>This award-winning site is both practical and informative

Resources and games

Word Pool

www.wordpool.co.uk

>An excellent site for book reviews, children's literature, writers and aspiring writers.

Crossbow Education

www.crossboweducation.com

>This is an excellent site full of resources, information and links to other sites.

Barrington Stoke

www.barringtonstoke.co.uk

>This is the site for a book publisher that specialises in high interest books for struggling readers.

Waterstones

www.waterstones.co.uk

On the website you can download a guide to choosing books for dyslexic readers:

http://www.waterstones.com/wat/images/special/mag/
waterstones_dyslexia_action_guide.pdf

Wordshark

www.wordshark.co.uk

This is a truly excellent piece of software that I use on a daily basis with my pupils. It is very versatile and suitable for children from ages 5 to 16.

Nessy

www.nessy.com

This is also a great site for software for dyslexic children. They love the games and there is also a CD to help with touch-typing.

Phonics

Free Phonics Worksheets

www.free-phonics-worksheets.com

This site provides worksheets for: consonant and vowel recognition; initial consonant sounds; beginning and end blends; consonant digraphs; silent letters; long vowel sounds.

First School Years

www.firstschoolyears.com

Offers a good selection of resources, including worksheets and some interactive games.

Primary Resources

www.primaryresources.co.uk

Click on 'English' and then 'Word level' to find a good selection of worksheets and activities. They cover early phonics and alphabet work, plurals, tenses, prefixes/suffixes.

BBC Schools

www.bbc.co.uk/schools/wordsandpictures/phonics/

A mix of very good interactive games and worksheets covering most phonic phases.

www.bbc.co.uk/schools/ks1bitesize/literacy/

A very good selection of interactive games focusing on phonics and sentence construction. Each is split into medium/hard/really hard and all of them are short and fun.

ICT Games

www.ictgames.com/literacy.html

A great selection of games.

Phonics Play

www.phonicsplay.co.uk

A selection of mostly simple interactive games.

Phonics

http://www.northwood.org.uk/phonics.htm

Interactive games for a range of sounds. Each sound has a couple of interactive games and a clever spelling game.

Note: A selection of phonics and spelling apps is also available via *iTunes* and other sources.

10 Glossary

Adjective A word that describes a noun. For example: *The* **happy** *dog.*

Adverb A word that describes a verb. It tells us how the verb is being performed. For example: *She sang* **badly**.

Auditory To do with hearing.

Auditory discrimination The ability to distinguish differences or similarities between sounds. For example: to be able to hear the difference between **f**, **th** and **v**.

Auditory memory One of the two types of working memory. It is the ability to remember what we have heard.

Automaticity The ability to do something automatically without consciously thinking about it.

Base word An original word before any prefixes or suffixes have been added. For example: in the word **helpful**, the base word is **help**.

Blend The ability to run individual sounds together to make a word. For example: **c-a-t** blends to make **cat** and **ta-ble** blends to make **table**.

Closed syllable A syllable that ends with a consonant. It has a short vowel sound. For example: **tab**.

Consonant All the letters of the alphabet that are not vowels.

Digraph A digraph is two or more letters that join together to make one sound. For example: **sh** as in **shop** and **ee** as in **week**.

Grapheme The letter or letters that represent a sound.

Homophones Words that sound the same but are spelt differently. For example: **here** and **hear**.

Kinaesthetic To do with movement.

Letter string A spelling pattern. For example: ould in could, would, should.

Long-term memory The area of our memory where information is stored more permanently.

Mnemonic A way of remembering how to spell tricky words. For example: Ants Never Yawn = any.

Multisensory learning A way of learning that uses more than one of our senses. For example: using the visual, auditory and kinaesthetic senses all at the same time.

Noun A naming word for people, places or objects. For example: James, Solihull, computer.

Open syllable A syllable that ends with a vowel. The vowel sound is long. For example: he, ta, ro.

Phoneme A single speech sound. For example: top has three sounds, t, o and p.

Phonemic awareness The ability to hear the separate sounds in a word.

Phonics A method for teaching reading and spelling that relies on the link between a sound and the letters that represent it.

Prefix A letter or group of letters that are added to a base word to change its meaning.

Preposition A word used with a noun to show place, position, time or means, for example, at home, in school, by car.

Proof-reading A method of checking written work for any mistakes.

Regular final syllable Groups of letters that commonly occur at the end of a word and form a separate syllable. For example: ble in table, or tion in station.

Short-term memory The part of our memory that stores information temporarily. Also known as working memory.

Suffix A letter or group of letters added to the end of a base word to change its use or meaning.

Superlative The form of an adjective that expresses the most. For example: happiest, tallest.

Syllable A beat in a word. Every syllable has a vowel sound.

Verb An action word. For example: *sing, run, shout*.

Visual To do with sight.

Vowels The letters *a, e, i, o, u*. The letter *y* sometimes acts like a vowel.

Working memory The part of the memory that you use when you are doing a task. It is where you store information temporarily while you are using it to work something out.